LOW FODMAP Diet COOKBOOK

A 7-Day Stress Free Meal Plan To Relieve IBS Symptoms with Delicious Gut-Soothing Recipes

By
Brandon Herrera

Copyright © 2023 by Brandon Herrera - All rights reserved.

The content contained within this book may not be reproduced, duplicated or transmitted without direct written permission from the author or the publisher.

Under no circumstances will any blame or legal responsibility be held against the publisher, or author, for any damages, reparation, or monetary loss due to the information contained within this book. Either directly or indirectly. You are responsible for your own choices, actions, and results.

<u>Legal Notice:</u>

This book is copyright protected. This book is only for personal use. You cannot amend, distribute, sell, use, quote or paraphrase any part, or the content within this book, without the consent of the author or publisher.

<u>Disclaimer Notice:</u>

Please note the information contained within this document is for educational and entertainment purposes only. All effort has been executed to present accurate, up to date, and reliable, complete information. No warranties of any kind are declared or implied. Readers acknowledge that the author is not engaging in the rendering of legal, financial, medical or professional advice. The content within this book has been derived from various sources. Please consult a licensed professional before attempting any techniques outlined in this book.

By reading this document, the reader agrees that under no circumstances is the author responsible for any losses, direct or indirect, which are incurred as a result of the use of the information contained within this document, including, but not limited to, — errors, omissions, or inaccuracies.

Your Free Gift

As a way of saying thanks for your purchase, I'm offering a copy of our **Digestive Health Wellness Guide**: *The Ultimate Digestive Health Wellness Guide To Understanding Your Gut And Living A More Pain-Free Life* for FREE to you!

To get instant access just go to: **prestigebookgroup.com**

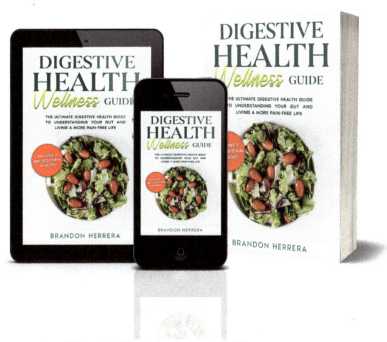

Inside this book you will discover:

- **14 Simple Tips** to improving your digestive health today
- How to prioritize these **4 mealtime habits** to get your digestive process working properly

- 5 of the most common forms of digestive health issues
- A quick gut health food checklist that *all dietitians* swear by
- And so much more!

If you want to conquer digestive health and live a more pain-free life, make sure to grab this free guide.

Table Of Contents

Your Free Gift 3

Introduction 7

Chapter 1: *FODMAPs and You* 9

What are Fodmaps? 10

Are Fodmaps a problem for you? (different types of problems: IBS-C & IBS-D, SIBO, Gluten) 11

Low Fodmap vs. Gluten Free 13

How do FODMAPs contribute to IBS symptoms? 14

What is the Low Fodmap Diet? 16

Who's the Low Fodmap Diet for? 17

Benefits of the Low Fodmap Diet 18

Key Chapter Takeaways 21

Chapter 2: *Your Gut and Food Relationship* 23

What is 'gut health'? 23

Gut reaction to food 24

How food can trigger gut symptoms 25

Understanding Triggers: The Secret Culprits (Onions And Garlic) 27

Key Chapter Takeaways 29

Chapter 3: *How to Follow a low FODMAP Diet* 30

Understanding How to Read Food Labels 30

Low FODMAPs staples for your pantry and fridge 33

Keeping Your Kitchen FODMAP Friendly 36

High FODMAP foods to avoid 37

Low FODMAP foods to eat 41

Different Drink Options for IBS 45

Cooking and Meal Planning 48

General Baking Practices 49

How to eat out on a low FODMAP diet 51

Key Chapter Takeaways 54

Chapter 4: *7-Day Low Fodmap Meal Plan* 56

Chapter 5: *Breakfast Recipes* 107

Chapter 6: *Lunch Recipes* 135

Chapter 7: *Dinner Recipes* 167

Conclusion 193

Resources 197

Introduction

Irritable Bowel Syndrome (IBS) is a condition that plagues nearly hundreds of thousands of people every year. What's even more unsettling is that there isn't a direct cure for IBS. Leaving many of us unequipped with the proper tools for combating IBS or any other digestive disorders.

We all know the struggles that come with irritable bowel syndrome. It's not a fun ride and it can sometimes interfere with our personal lives and our goals. It's as if our lives must be optimized around our gut health and going to the bathroom.

It all starts with a gut feeling (and I'm not talking about intuition). Sometimes that gut feeling feels like someone is wringing your colon like a wet towel. Or intense sharp pain in your abdomen that feels like your stomach has been pierced with a knife.

It's also not ideal to go 3-4 days without having a *movement*. Sometimes when that movement does come, you end up pushing harder than you've ever pushed in your life feeling as if you're on the brink of giving birth! All for just a few little rock pebbles. Doesn't sound like a fair trade, does it?

On top of that, you've completely run out of toilet paper. Happy trails.

All jokes aside, living with IBS and other digestive disorders only complicates our lives.

Take it from someone who has suffered with digestive issues for many years. I could never quite figure out what was causing my issues. Was it the food I was eating? Was it my busy schedule and not finding time to use the bathroom? Stress? Too much coffee? It wasn't until I took a full inventory of the foods I was eating to fix my digestive issues.

As it turns out, many of the foods I've come to love and enjoy *(like bread for example)* are rich in what turned out to be the culprit - *gluten.*

Gluten just so happens to be for me, what kryptonite is to Superman.

It's a combination of bad and ugly for my gut health. Fortunately, by applying many of the principles, guidelines, and recipes that are in this exact Low Fodmap Diet Cookbook, I was able to quickly turn things around for the better!

I'm happy to help you do the same in this book.

-Chapter 1-
FODMAPs and You

Living with Irritable Bowel Syndrome (IBS) can be a daily challenge, affecting your digestive system and overall well-being. The constant discomfort, bloating, unpredictable bowel movements, and dietary restrictions make it feel like your digestive system is playing a never-ending game of roulette. However, there is hope. The low FODMAP diet, a scientifically backed approach, has been shown to relieve and help manage IBS symptoms effectively.

To effectively combat any problem, it's essential to understand its roots. IBS is a complex gastrointestinal disorder that affects millions of people worldwide. It can manifest in various ways, causing abdominal pain, bloating, gas, diarrhea, or constipation. While the exact causes of IBS remain somewhat elusive, research suggests that multiple factors, including genetic predisposition, food passing through your gut too quickly or too slowly, and oversensitive nerves in your gut could be the cause.

What are Fodmaps?

FODMAP is an acronym that represents "fermentable oligo-, di-, and monosaccharides and polyols." These substances consist of short-chain carbohydrates that cannot be fully digested and have an osmotic effect, drawing water into the digestive tract.

- **Fermentable**: Fermentable foods serve as a fuel source for your gut bacteria. They convert them to gases by undergoing a chemical process called fermentation.

- **Oligosaccharides**: Oligosaccharides refers to soluble plant fibers known as prebiotics, which nourish beneficial bacteria in your gut. Foods such as onions, garlic, wheat, rye, nuts, artichokes, beans/lentils, and certain wheat products contain oligosaccharides. Sensitivity to oligosaccharides may explain some cases of non-celiac gluten sensitivity. It's worth noting that gluten-free grains have lower levels of fermentable sugars than grains containing gluten, so if you are sensitive to gluten, you may react to the oligosaccharides in wheat products.

- **Disaccharides**: Disaccharides consist of lactose-containing products such as milk, yogurt, soft cheese, ice cream, buttermilk, condensed milk, and whipped cream. Lactose intolerance is a common food intolerance.

- **Monosaccharides**: Monosaccharides refer to fructose, the fermentable sugar found in fruits such as watermelon, apples, pears, and mango, and sweeteners such as agave nectar, honey, and high fructose corn syrup. However, not all fruits are equally affected, as it depends on the quantities and proportions of fructose present.

- **Polyols**: Polyols are sugar alcohols commonly used as artificial sweeteners. They include xylitol and isomalt in low-calorie sweeteners, such as those in sugar-free gum and mints. They can also occur naturally in certain fruits, such as mannitol and sorbitol in apples, pears, cauliflower, stone fruits, mushrooms, and snow peas.

Due to their indigestible nature, these carbohydrates are fermented by the bacteria in the gut, leading to increased gas and the production of short-chain fatty acids.

According to the National Library of Medicine (NLM), approximately 60% of individuals with irritable bowel syndrome (IBS) have reported that these carbohydrates can either cause or worsen their symptoms.

Consequently, FODMAPs are well-known for their ability to trigger digestive symptoms, including bloating, gas, stomach pain, and changes in bowel habits, such as constipation, diarrhea, or a combination of both.

Are Fodmaps a problem for you? (different types of problems: IBS-C & IBS-D, SIBO, Gluten)

FODMAPs can be problematic for certain people, particularly those who experience gastrointestinal issues like irritable bowel syndrome with constipation (IBS-C), irritable bowel syndrome with diarrhea (IBS-D), small intestinal bacterial overgrowth (SIBO), or gluten sensitivities. Let's take a closer look at how FODMAPs can contribute to these problems:

- **Irritable bowel syndrome (IBS)**: For people with IBS, FODMAPs can trigger symptoms like bloating, gas, abdominal pain, diarrhea, or constipation. These carbohydrates are not fully absorbed in the small intestine. When they reach the large intestine, they can be fermented by gut bacteria, producing gas and causing discomfort. A low-FODMAP diet can help alleviate these symptoms and improve the overall quality of life for people with IBS.

- **IBS-C:** For people with IBS-C, the low-FODMAP diet can help reduce symptoms such as abdominal discomfort, bloating, and constipation. High-FODMAP foods can lead to increased water content in the intestine, causing bloating and worsening constipation symptoms in susceptible individuals.

- **IBS-D**: The low-FODMAP diet can also provide relief for individuals with IBS-D. High-FODMAP foods are rapidly fermented by gut bacteria, leading to increased gas production and water retention in the intestines, resulting in diarrhea and abdominal pain. By reducing FODMAP intake, these symptoms can often be alleviated.

- **Small intestinal bacterial overgrowth (SIBO):** SIBO is a condition where there is an abnormal increase in bacteria in the small intestine. These bacteria can ferment

FODMAPs, leading to symptoms such as bloating, gas, diarrhea, and abdominal pain. A low-FODMAP diet can help reduce the intake of fermentable carbohydrates, potentially reducing symptoms for people with SIBO.

- **Gluten sensitivity**: It's important to note that FODMAPs differ from gluten. Gluten is a protein found in wheat, barley, and rye, while FODMAPs refer to certain types of carbohydrates. However, some people with non-celiac gluten sensitivity may mistakenly attribute their symptoms to gluten when it could be the FODMAP content in their foods. In such cases, a low-FODMAP diet can help identify the true triggers of their symptoms.

Low Fodmap vs. Gluten Free

The main difference between a low-FODMAP diet and a gluten-free diet lies in the components they restrict and the conditions they address. Here's a breakdown:

- **Low-FODMAP diet**: The low-FODMAP diet focuses on reducing or eliminating certain carbohydrates called FODMAPs. The low-FODMAP diet is primarily used to manage irritable bowel syndrome (IBS) symptoms and other functional gastrointestinal disorders. It involves eliminating high-FODMAP foods for some time, followed by a systematic reintroduction process to identify individual trigger foods.

- **Gluten-free diet**: A Gluten-Free diet involves avoiding all sources of gluten, a protein found in wheat, barley, rye, and their derivatives. This includes products like bread, pasta, cereals, baked goods, and many processed foods that contain gluten ingredients.

People with celiac disease, an autoimmune disorder triggered by gluten, must strictly follow a gluten-free diet to avoid intestinal damage and associated symptoms. In addition to celiac disease, some individuals may have non-celiac gluten sensitivity and experience symptoms similar to celiac disease without the characteristic intestinal damage. For these individuals, following a gluten-free diet may provide symptom relief.

A strict gluten-free diet is a lifelong requirement for people with celiac disease to maintain gut health and prevent complications. However, individuals with non-celiac gluten sensitivity may find that reducing or avoiding gluten can relieve their symptoms, but the diet duration may vary for each person.

How do FODMAPs contribute to IBS symptoms?

FODMAPs can contribute to Irritable Bowel Syndrome (IBS) symptoms in several ways:

- **Poor absorption**: FODMAPs are a group of carbohydrates that are not fully absorbed in the small intestine.

Instead, they pass into the large intestine, where they can draw water into the bowel and be fermented by gut bacteria. This fermentation produces gas, leading to bloating, distension, and abdominal discomfort.

- **Increased water content:** FODMAPs have an osmotic effect, attracting water into the intestine. This increased water content can result in looser or more frequent bowel movements, contributing to diarrhea in individuals with IBS-D (IBS with diarrhea).

- **Gut sensitivity:** Some individuals with IBS may have heightened gut sensitivity or altered sensory processing in the digestive system. FODMAPs can stimulate the gut and cause discomfort or pain in sensitive individuals.

- **Changes in gut motility**: FODMAPs can influence the movement of the intestines. In some people with IBS, FODMAPs may accelerate or slow down gut motility, leading to symptoms of diarrhea or constipation.

- **Interaction with gut bacteria:** FODMAPs serve as a food source for gut bacteria. In individuals with an imbalanced gut microbiota, the fermentation of FODMAPs can produce excessive gas and other byproducts, contributing to gut symptoms.

What is the Low Fodmap Diet?

The low-FODMAP diet is specifically designed to help people with irritable bowel syndrome (IBS) have improved control over their symptoms by restricting certain foods.

The Low FODMAP diet aims to reduce the intake of these troublesome carbohydrates, relieving IBS symptoms. It allows the gut to heal and reduces the overall burden on the digestive system. It consists of three phases: restriction, reintroduction, and personalization.

- **Restriction** - During this phase, restrict or limit the consumption of high-FODMAP foods for two to six weeks. This allows your body to reset and provides a baseline for understanding your triggers. The duration can be determined by your doctor, considering your symptoms, health history, and current dietary patterns.

- **Reintroduction** - Gradually reintroduce high-FODMAP foods back into your diet, one food at a time, for three days for each food. As you introduce new foods, pay close attention to any changes or reactions in your IBS symptoms.

- **Personalization** - Customize your diet to suit your needs based on the information gathered during the reintroduction phase. Identify and avoid high-FODMAP foods that trigger or worsen your IBS symptoms. At the same time, incorporate other high-FODMAP foods that were well-tolerated during the reintroduction process. This personalized approach aims to optimize your diet while managing your IBS symptoms effectively.

Who's the Low Fodmap Diet for?

A low-FODMAP diet plan isn't for everyone, but it can benefit people who experience irritable bowel syndrome (IBS) symptoms, small intestinal bacterial overgrowth (SIBO), and other gastrointestinal disorders. This is because most FODMAPs serve as prebiotics, promoting the growth of beneficial bacteria in your gut. Eliminating these substances may have a negative impact on the balance of intestinal bacteria, which directly influences your overall health.

Furthermore, excluding various fruits and vegetables from your diet can result in essential vitamin and mineral deficiencies. Additionally, it may significantly reduce your dietary fiber intake, which could worsen constipation.

Here are some groups of people who might benefit from a low-FODMAP diet plan:

- **Individuals with IBS**: IBS is a common gastrointestinal disorder characterized by recurring abdominal pain, bloating, and changes in bowel habits. Research has shown that a low-FODMAP diet can help alleviate symptoms in people with IBS.

- **Other functional gastrointestinal disorders**: Besides IBS, conditions such as functional bloating, diarrhea, and constipation may also benefit from a low-FODMAP diet.

- **Those with diagnosed food intolerances:** Some people may have specific intolerances to certain FODMAPs, such as lactose or fructose intolerance. In such cases, a low-FODMAP diet can help identify trigger foods and manage symptoms.

- **Athletes or individuals seeking short-term digestive relief:** Some athletes or people about to participate in high-intensity events may follow a low-FODMAP diet for a short period to reduce gastrointestinal distress during exercise.

Benefits of the Low Fodmap Diet

The low-FODMAP diet has been shown to provide several benefits for people with certain gastrointestinal conditions. Here are some potential benefits of following a low-FODMAP diet:

- **Symptom relief for IBS**: The primary benefit of a low-FODMAP diet is the reduction of symptoms associated with irritable bowel syndrome (IBS). Many people with IBS experience bloating, gas, abdominal pain, diarrhea, or constipation, and following a low-FODMAP diet can help alleviate these symptoms in many cases.

- **Identification of trigger foods**: People can identify specific triggers that worsen their symptoms by eliminating high-FODMAP foods and then systematically reintroducing them. This personalized approach allows people to create a customized diet plan that avoids the specific FODMAPs that trigger their symptoms, leading to better management of their condition.

- **Improved quality of life:** IBS symptoms can significantly impact an individual's quality of life, affecting daily activities, social interactions, and overall well-being. By reducing or eliminating symptoms through a low-FODMAP diet, people often experience an improvement in their quality of life. They are better able to engage in their usual activities without discomfort.

- **Relief for other gastrointestinal disorders:** While the low-FODMAP diet was initially developed for IBS, it has shown promise in helping manage symptoms of other functional gastrointestinal disorders, such as functional bloating, diarrhea, and constipation. Some individuals with these conditions may also experience symptom relief by following a low-FODMAP diet.

- **Better dietary diversity**: While the elimination phase of the low-FODMAP diet restricts certain high-FODMAP foods, it encourages the inclusion of low-FODMAP alternatives. This can increase dietary diversity as individuals explore and incorporate a wider range of low-FODMAP fruits, vegetables, grains, proteins, and fats into their meals.

- **May reduce digestive symptoms:** The symptoms of irritable bowel syndrome (IBS) can greatly differ but commonly involve stomach pain, bloating, reflux, flatulence, and urgency in bowel movements. These symptoms can significantly impact one's quality of life.

  Research has demonstrated that adopting a low FODMAP diet can reduce both stomach pain and bloating. Evidence from four studies has consistently shown that following a low FODMAP diet increases the likelihood of alleviating stomach pain by 81% and bloating by 75%.

  Furthermore, several other studies support these findings and indicate that this dietary approach can also help manage symptoms of flatulence, diarrhea, and constipation associated with IBS.

- **Reduced Histamine:** Histamine is a potent inflammatory signal crucial in allergic reactions and various immune responses. Certain foods naturally contain histamine, while consuming certain other foods can potentially stimulate the release of histamine in the body.

Key Chapter Takeaways

- Irritable Bowel Syndrome (IBS) is a complex gastrointestinal disorder affecting millions worldwide, causing symptoms like abdominal pain, bloating, gas, and changes in bowel movements.

- FODMAPs (fermentable oligo-, di-, and monosaccharides and polyols) are short-chain carbohydrates that cannot be fully digested and can trigger digestive symptoms in individuals with IBS. They are found in various foods, including fruits, vegetables, grains, and dairy products.

- FODMAPs can be problematic for people with IBS, IBS with constipation (IBS-C), IBS with diarrhea (IBS-D), small intestinal bacterial overgrowth (SIBO), and gluten sensitivities. Restricting FODMAP intake through a low-FODMAP diet can help alleviate symptoms in these individuals.

- The low-FODMAP diet comprises three phases: restriction, reintroduction, and personalization. During the restriction phase, high-FODMAP foods are limited for a few weeks. In the reintroduction phase, foods are gradually reintroduced to identify individual triggers. A customized diet is created based on the identified triggers in the personalization phase.

- Research has shown that following a low-FODMAP diet can reduce symptoms such as stomach pain, bloating, flatulence, diarrhea, and constipation associated with IBS. It may also help reduce histamine levels and manage symptoms of other gastrointestinal disorders.

- Benefits of the Low FODMAP Diet include symptom relief for IBS, identification of trigger foods, improved quality of life, relief for other gastrointestinal disorders, enhanced dietary diversity, and reduced digestive symptoms like stomach pain, bloating, and flatulence. Additionally, it may help reduce histamine levels in the body.

-Chapter 2-
Your Gut and Food Relationship

We've all experienced a "gut feeling," although this popular phrase is rooted in intuition and instinct, our gut genuinely influences our well-being and overall functioning.

In recent years, "gut health" has emerged as a trending concept. The term refers to the intricate ecosystem of microbes and their genetic material residing in our gastrointestinal tract, known as the gut microbiome. Extensive research has revealed the profound impact of gut bacteria on various aspects of our health, encompassing digestion and our mental well-being.

What is 'gut health'?

Our digestive system, commonly known as the "gut," is an intricate network of tissues and organs working together to break down and absorb the food we consume. This system includes essential components such as the mouth, esophagus, stomach, pancreas, gallbladder, liver, small intestine, and large intestine.

Within the gut, an extraordinary community of microorganisms known as the microbiota thrives. This community consists of approximately 500 known species, predominantly composed of bacteria, yeast, fungi, and viruses. Remarkably, each individual carries around 100 trillion of these microbes, primarily in the digestive tract. However, microbial communities can also be found in other areas of the body, including the nose, skin, and mouth.

Emerging research suggests that the microbiota, along with its collection of genomes collectively called the microbiome, may exert a profound influence on our health, potentially rivaling the impact of our inherited genes.

Gut reaction to food

Gut reactions to food can be categorized into immunological and non-immunological reactions. Let's define both terms:

- **Immunological reactions:** Immunological reactions involve the immune system's response to specific components in food. These reactions are typically mediated by antibodies, specifically immunoglobulin E (IgE), and are referred to as IgE-mediated food allergies. When a person with a food allergy consumes an allergenic food, their immune system recognizes the food as harmful and triggers an allergic response. Symptoms can range from mild to severe and may include hives, itching, swelling, difficulty breathing, gastrointestinal distress, and in severe cases, anaphylaxis. Immunological reactions are relatively rare but can be life-threatening. They require strict avoidance of allergenic food and often necessitate medical management.

- **Non-immunological reactions**: Non-immunological reactions to food do not involve the immune system's response. These reactions are more commonly seen and can have various causes.

How food can trigger gut symptoms

Food can trigger gut symptoms in several ways, particularly in people with gastrointestinal conditions or sensitivities. Here are some mechanisms through which food can contribute to gut symptoms:

- **Food intolerances:** Some people have specific intolerances to certain components of food. For example, lactose intolerance is the inability to digest lactose, a sugar found in dairy products. Similarly, some people may have intolerances to gluten, fructose, or other substances. Consuming foods containing these substances can lead to symptoms such as bloating, gas, abdominal pain, and diarrhea.

- **Allergies and sensitivities**: Food allergies and sensitivities involve an immune system response to specific proteins in food. In allergic reactions, the immune system identifies certain food proteins as harmful, triggering an allergic response that can include gastrointestinal symptoms such as abdominal pain, vomiting, or diarrhea. Food sensitivities may produce similar symptoms, but the immune response is less severe or immediate.

- **Gut inflammation**: Some foods, especially those high in saturated fats, refined sugars, and processed ingredients, can promote inflammation in the gut. Inflammation can contribute to gut symptoms and worsen conditions such as inflammatory bowel disease (IBD) or leaky gut syndrome.

- **Gut-brain axis**: The gut and brain are closely connected through the gut-brain axis, allowing communication between the digestive and central nervous systems. Emotional factors like stress, anxiety, or excitement can trigger gut symptoms or worsen existing symptoms. This is often seen in individuals with IBS, where stress and emotions can influence gut motility and sensitivity.

- **Imbalance in gut microbiota**: The gut microbiota refers to the community of microorganisms residing in the digestive tract. An imbalance in the gut microbiota, such as an overgrowth of certain bacteria or a reduction in beneficial bacteria, can contribute to gut symptoms. Certain foods, such as highly processed or sugary foods, can negatively impact the gut microbiota, promoting the growth of harmful bacteria and potentially leading to symptoms like bloating, gas, or altered bowel movements.

- **Inflammatory bowel disease (IBD):** Conditions like Crohn's disease and ulcerative colitis involve chronic inflammation in the digestive tract. Certain foods can trigger or worsen inflammation, leading to abdominal pain, diarrhea, and other symptoms.

Understanding Triggers: The Secret Culprits (Onions And Garlic)

Onions and garlic, while widely used in cooking and loved for their flavor, can be considered "secret culprits" when it comes to triggering gut symptoms for some individuals. Here's why:

- **High FODMAP content**: Onions and garlic belong to a group of vegetables known as alliums. Alliums contain high amounts of FODMAPs, specifically fructans, a carbohydrate type that can be poorly absorbed in the small intestine. In individuals with irritable bowel syndrome (IBS) or other conditions sensitive to FODMAPs, consuming onions and garlic can lead to symptoms such as bloating, gas, abdominal pain, and altered bowel movements. It's worth noting that the FODMAP content can vary depending on the type and preparation of onions and garlic (e.g., raw vs. cooked).

- **Fructans and gut bacteria:** The fructans present in onions, and garlic can reach the undigested large intestine, serving as a food source for gut bacteria. This fermentation process can produce gas, leading to bloating and discomfort. Additionally, the byproducts of fermentation can affect the water content and movement in the intestine, potentially causing diarrhea or constipation in susceptible individuals.

- **Sensitivities and intolerances**: Some people may have specific sensitivities or intolerances to certain components found in onions and garlic. For example, some people may be sensitive to the organosulfur compounds responsible for the pungent odor and taste of these vegetables. These compounds can irritate the digestive system and trigger symptoms in susceptible individuals, even without FODMAP-related issues.

Key Chapter Takeaways

- Gut health refers to the ecosystem of microbes in our gastrointestinal tract, known as the gut microbiome, which profoundly impacts our health.

- The gut consists of a complex network of tissues and organs involved in digestion, with the microbiota being the community of microorganisms residing in the gut.

- Gut reactions to food can be immunological (involving the immune system's response) or non-immunological.

- Food can trigger gut symptoms through food intolerances, allergies, inflammation, gut-brain axis, imbalances in gut microbiota, and conditions like inflammatory bowel disease (IBD).

- High in FODMAPs (fructans), onions, and garlic can trigger gut symptoms for individuals with sensitivities or conditions like IBS due to poor absorption, fermentation, and potential intolerances.

-Chapter 3-
How to Follow a low FODMAP Diet

Following a low FODMAP diet can be a helpful approach for IBS. By understanding and implementing these principles, you can better control your digestive symptoms and make informed choices about the foods you consume.

Understanding How to Read Food Labels

Reading food labels carefully is crucial when following a low-FODMAP diet to identify potential high-FODMAP ingredients or additives. Here are some tips to help you navigate food labels effectively:

- **Check the ingredient list**: Review the ingredient list on the food label. Look for ingredients that are known as high-FODMAP foods or ingredients that contain high-FODMAP components. Common high-FODMAP ingredients include onions, garlic, wheat, barley, rye, honey, and high-fructose corn syrup.

- **Look for hidden sources of FODMAPs**: Some ingredients may contain FODMAPs but might not be explicitly mentioned on the label. Look out for terms like "natural flavors," "spices," or "artificial sweeteners," as these can sometimes include FODMAP-containing ingredients. If you're unsure about a particular ingredient, do some research or consult a registered dietitian for clarification.

- **Pay attention to serving sizes**: Serving sizes on food labels can significantly impact the FODMAP content of food. A small amount of high-FODMAP food may be considered low FODMAP if the serving size is small enough. Know the recommended serving size and adjust your portion accordingly.

- **Be cautious of additive ingredients:** Some additives, such as certain emulsifiers, stabilizers, and thickeners, can be high in FODMAPs. Examples include inulin, fructo-oligosaccharides (FOS), and polyols like sorbitol and mannitol. These ingredients can be found in processed foods, sauces, dressings, and certain low-calorie or sugar-free products. Check for their presence on the ingredient list and avoid products that contain these additives if you are sensitive to them.

- **Look for low-FODMAP certifications or labels:** Some food products specifically indicate that they are suitable for a low-FODMAP diet by including a certification or label from FODMAP-friendly organizations. These products have undergone testing to ensure their FODMAP content is within acceptable limits. Keep an eye out for such labels if you prefer pre-packaged foods.

- **Be careful with "no added" claims**: "No added" claims (e.g., "no added onions" or "no added garlic") don't necessarily mean the product is low in FODMAPs. These claims only indicate that the specific ingredient hasn't been added separately, but there might still be traces or derivatives of the ingredient present. Always check the ingredients list to ensure there are no high-FODMAP ingredients.

- **Keep a list of safe and trigger foods**: As you learn about FODMAPs and your triggers, maintain a list. This can serve as a quick reference when reading food labels and making purchasing decisions.

- **Consider cross-contamination**: In some cases, cross-contamination of FODMAPs can occur during food processing or manufacturing. This is particularly relevant for products processed in facilities that handle high-FODMAP ingredients. If you have severe sensitivities or strict dietary requirements, you may want to contact the manufacturer or choose products with dedicated gluten-free or low FODMAP certifications.

Low FODMAPs staples for your pantry and fridge

Navigating the low FODMAP diet can be challenging and time-consuming, particularly when planning and preparing meals. However, you can simplify the process and save valuable time by stocking your pantry with these essential staples. These items will make following the low FODMAP diet more manageable and serve as a lifesaver during busy weeks.

- **Protein sources:** Choose not marinated or breaded meats, poultry, fish, and seafood, as well as eggs, tempeh, firm tofu, well-rinsed canned legumes (1/4 cup), and most seeds and nuts (except cashews and pistachios).

- **Dairy products and/or substitutes:** Opt for lactose-free milk and yogurt, firm cheeses, and soy beverages (only if made from protein or fortified almonds).

- **Grain products**: Imagine a world without pasta, and it's a world I'd rather not live in. Pasta is a versatile and time-saving staple to keep in your pantry for those hectic weeks. Fortunately, fantastic wheat-free alternatives are available, such as brown rice, corn, and quinoa pasta. These alternatives satisfy your pasta cravings and provide an extra protein boost compared to traditional wheat pasta. If you want to amp up the protein content, add ingredients like chicken, ground beef, or even sprinkle some nutrient-rich hemp seeds. Other grain products include cereals, breads, and crackers made from rice, quinoa, oats, millet, and buckwheat.

- **Vegetables**: Include eggplant, bell pepper, bok choy, carrot, cucumber, lettuce, potato, spinach, tomato, and zucchini.

- **Fruits**: Enjoy blueberries, cantaloupe, clementine, kiwi, oranges, raspberries, strawberries, and tangerines.

- **Seasonings**: Enhance your meals with miso, mustard, soy sauce, spices, and vinegar.

- **Low FODMAP Bars:** Having convenient snack bars can be a lifesaver when you're constantly on the move due to work or family events. These bars provide a portable and satisfying option to keep hunger at bay and prevent the need to grab something hastily that could potentially trigger symptoms.

- **Peanut Butter**: Peanut butter is an excellent choice among low FODMAP nut kinds of butter since you can enjoy a satisfying portion of 2 tablespoons. While the brand isn't crucial, organic and all-natural peanut butter is recommended. Ensure that the ingredients list solely includes peanuts and perhaps a small amount of salt. Certain grocery stores even offer the convenience of freshly ground peanut butter, which presents a fantastic alternative worth considering.

- **Gluten-Free All-Purpose Flour:** If you are passionate about baking, it's wise to have a 1-to-1 gluten-free all-purpose flour readily available in your pantry. While they may not be flawless substitutes, they offer a viable option for your baking needs.

- **Pure Maple Syrup**: Did you enjoy adding honey to everything before starting the low FODMAP diet? Don't worry; you don't have to miss out on that delightful touch of sweetness for your oats, teas, baked goods, dressings, and marinades. Simply replace it with pure maple syrup and enjoy the same flavorful experience.

- **Salsa**: Salsa is an essential pantry and fridge staple, as it adds a burst of flavor to a wide variety of dishes! Whether you're making tacos, huevos rancheros, shredded chicken, or simply looking for a tasty snack, having a low FODMAP salsa on hand is a must.

- **Garlic Infused Olive Oil:** What aroma is more enticing than the scent of fresh garlic sizzling in a pan? Unfortunately, using regular garlic can be troublesome for those following a low FODMAP diet. Low Fodmap Garlic-infused olive oil is the perfect solution to infuse your dishes with that same delightful flavor and aromatic experience while avoiding unwanted digestive discomfort. Enjoy the taste and aroma of garlic without the side effects by incorporating Low fodmap garlic-infused olive oil into your culinary creations.

Keeping Your Kitchen FODMAP Friendly

- **Stock up on compliant starches:** Starches are particularly economical when considering affordable food choices, especially when purchased in larger quantities. On the low-FODMAP diet, you can enjoy budget-friendly options such as russet potatoes, sweet potatoes, squash, oats, quinoa, and brown rice.

  These food options can be cost-effective and serve as excellent sources of fiber, protein, and various essential nutrients, making them beneficial additions to your diet.

- **Always have something prepped in advance:** Certain weight loss diets acknowledge the possibility of occasional slip-ups. While you may occasionally veer off the low-FODMAP path, proper meal prepping can significantly increase your chances of success.

  In times of uncertainty, having readily available low-FODMAP foods in your refrigerator can be a lifesaver, particularly when time is limited. Preparing certain foods in larger quantities, such as oatmeal, baked potatoes, sautéed veggies, and grilled protein sources, can be incredibly helpful.

  Adopting this practice will motivate you to adhere to the low-FODMAP diet while minimizing the temptation that may arise from other food options around you.

- **Rotate your fruits and veggies:** When managing expenses, purchasing fresh produce can often be expensive. Opting to shop in the frozen section or farmer's markets can provide you with better deals and value for your money. Additionally, embracing seasonal produce can be a more economical approach to stocking up on vegetables.

While the low-FODMAP diet suggests limited fruit consumption, it encourages the inclusion of a diverse range of vegetables. It's beneficial to vary your vegetable selection each week. For instance, if you prepared steamed carrots, bok choy, and cabbage one week, consider incorporating eggplant, kale, and green beans into your meals the following week.

This approach maintains your interest in the food you consume and ensures that you receive a wide array of nutrients despite the dietary restrictions imposed by the low-FODMAP protocol.

High FODMAP foods to avoid

Please note that the following list does not encompass every single food to avoid when following a Low FODMAP Diet.

VEGETABLES

- Garlic, garlic salt, garlic powder, pickled garlic - avoid entirely
- Onions, onion powder, pickled onions - avoid entirely if possible

- Artichoke
- Asparagus
- Broccoli
- Brussels sprouts
- Cabbage
- Cauliflower
- Green and yellow beans
- Leeks
- Mushrooms
- Sugar snap peas
- Summer squash

FRUITS

Some fruit can be high in fructose, so it's best to avoid eating any kind of fruit.

- Apples, applesauce, apple juice
- Apricots
- Avocados
- Bananas
- Blackberries
- Canned fruit in fruit juice
- Cherries
- Dried fruit (raisins, currants, dates, figs, prunes)
- Fruit juice
- Grapes
- Lychee
- Mango

- Nectarines
- Peaches
- Pears
- Pineapples
- Plums
- Watermelon

BEANS AND LEGUMES

- Beans
- Black-eyed peas
- Chickpeas
- Lentils
- Lima beans
- Kidney beans, cannellini beans
- Pinto beans
- Soybeans
- Split peas

MEAT, POULTRY, AND SEAFOOD

It is advisable to steer clear of marinated or processed meats that often contain high-FODMAP ingredients like garlic and onion. Therefore, it is recommended to avoid the following:

- Marinated meat, poultry, or seafood
- Sausages and salami
- Some processed meats

DAIRY AND DAIRY ALTERNATIVES

- Cow, goat, and sheep milk and milk products
- Coconut milk
- Custard
- Ice cream
- Soft un-ripened cheeses and fresh cheeses —brie, cottage cheese, cream cheese, ricotta, sour cream
- Soy milk
- Yogurt

GRAINS

To make informed dietary choices, it is crucial to carefully examine food labels and abstain from consuming bread, cereals, pasta, cookies, snack bars, and pastries that are made with the following ingredients:

- Barley
- Rye
- Wheat

NUTS

- Cashews
- Pistachios

SWEETENERS

- Agave
- High fructose corn syrup
- Honey

SUGAR SUBSTITUTES

Avoid many sugar-free gums and candies containing these sugar substitutes:

- Isomalt
- Lactitol
- Maltitol
- Mannitol
- Sorbitol
- Xylitol

FIBER SUPPLEMENTS

- Inulin

BEVERAGES

- Beer
- Chamomile, chia, dandelion, fennel, and oolong tea
- Port
- Rosé wine
- Sherry
- Soft drinks made with high-fructose corn syrup

Low FODMAP foods to eat

While following a low-FODMAP diet, you can include the following foods in your meals. Please note that this is not an exhaustive list.

VEGETABLES

- Bell peppers
- Bok choy
- Carrots
- Celery
- Chives
- Cucumber
- Eggplant
- Green beans
- Kale
- Lettuce
- Potatoes
- Pumpkin
- Radishes
- Spinach
- Tomatoes
- Winter squash
- Yams
- Zucchini
- Artichoke
- Ginger
- Sweet potato
- Olives
- Potato

FRUITS

- Blueberries

- Cantaloupe
- Grapefruit
- Kiwi
- Lemons
- Limes
- Papaya
- Passion fruit
- Pineapple (limit)
- Raspberries
- Strawberries
- Star anise
- Orange
- Honeydew melon

MEAT, POULTRY, AND SEAFOOD

- Plain cooked meat: beef, chicken, lamb, pork, turkey
- Canned fish (check ingredients)
- Fresh fish and seafood
- Frozen fish and seafood (as long as nothing else is added)

DAIRY, DAIRY ALTERNATIVES, AND EGGS

- Almond milk
- Eggs
- Aged hard cheeses
- Cashew milk
- Lactose-free milk
- Lactose-free yogurt
- Rice milk

NUTS AND SEEDS

- Almond butter
- Macadamia nuts
- Peanuts
- Seeds
- Walnuts

BREAD, CEREALS, AND PASTA

- Bread, pasta, cereal, pastries, and flours made from corn, potato, rice, oats, quinoa, or spelt

SWEETENERS AND SWEETS

- Dark chocolate
- Maple syrup
- Table sugar (sucrose)
- Rice malt syrup

SUGAR SUBSTITUTES

- Aspartame
- Saccharin
- Sucralose

Different Drink Options for IBS

Soft Drinks

Sodas may not be the best choice for individuals with IBS due to carbonation, which can lead to excessive gassiness and discomfort. Taking care of your overall health is important, and reducing or eliminating sodas can be a step in the right direction.

Regular sodas contain high levels of sugar, which have been linked to obesity, diabetes, and heart disease. Meanwhile, diet sodas, often containing artificial sweeteners, have also been associated with weight gain and may not be ideal for those with sensitive digestive systems.

A refreshing alternative to sodas is iced tea. Whether you prefer black, green, white, or herbal teas beneficial for IBS, iced tea can be satisfying. You can easily prepare a pitcher of homemade iced tea to keep in the refrigerator or opt for unsweetened iced tea when dining out. Add a small amount of sugar to your tea instead of artificial sweeteners if desired. In moderation, this should not typically trigger symptoms and allows you to enjoy a flavorful beverage.

Probiotic Drinks

Incorporating fermented drinks into your diet can be a beneficial choice for individuals with IBS. These drinks can positively impact the composition of gut bacteria, potentially leading to a reduction in symptoms.

Fermented drinks, such as kombucha, kefir, and yogurt drinks, contain a variety of probiotic strains that promote gut health. Kombucha, a fermented tea, can be enjoyed by selecting a low-sugar option. It's important to read the label to ensure it doesn't have a high sugar content. It's worth noting that kombucha naturally contains a small amount of alcohol.

Kefir, a fermented milk drink, undergoes a fermentation process that significantly reduces lactose content, making it suitable for lactose intolerant individuals. Non-dairy alternatives like coconut kefirs are also available for those who prefer dairy-free options.

Yogurt drinks are another choice to consider. Checking the labels and avoiding varieties with excessive added sugars is essential. Choose yogurt drinks without high-FODMAP fruits to prevent potential digestive discomfort.

Green Juices

Green juices are prepared using a juicer, which extracts the liquid from fruits and vegetables, leaving behind most of the pulp. This process results in a juice that contains less insoluble fiber, which can be harder to digest.

Drinking green juices allows you to consume fruits and vegetables more rapidly and in higher concentrations than eating them whole. As a result, you can quickly benefit from a concentrated infusion of phytonutrients while obtaining a good amount of soluble fiber that is more tolerable for people with IBS.

Green Smoothies

Green smoothies are deliciously blended beverages that combine liquids, vegetables, and fruits into a nutritious concoction.

You'll need a high-powered blender capable of thoroughly blending leafy greens to create a green smoothie. Start by blending the greens with a liquid base before incorporating other ingredients.

Choose low-FODMAP greens and fruits when selecting your ingredients. Spinach is a nice and versatile green, to begin with.

For added sweetness, bananas are a fantastic choice, while berries provide an excellent source of phytonutrients. Avoid blackberries as they have higher FODMAP levels.

Add a dollop of nut butter, a spoonful of coconut oil, or half an avocado to incorporate healthy anti-inflammatory fats. Chia seeds and ground flaxseed are additional options that can aid in managing IBS symptoms.

When choosing a liquid for your smoothie, consider:

- Almond milk (in small quantities)
- Coconut milk (up to 1/2 cup)
- Coconut water (limited to 3 ounces)
- Kefir
- Lactose-free milk

- Rice milk
- Water

These options provide a variety of flavors and textures to enhance your green smoothie experience.

Cooking and Meal Planning

Proper planning is essential for achieving success on the low-FODMAP diet. This entails ensuring your fridge and pantry are well-stocked with the right food items. While certain foods like baby carrots and bananas can be conveniently enjoyed as grab-and-go options, others may require some preparation.

Cook your foods in batches

Maximize your time and effort by preparing large batches of low-FODMAP foods. By dedicating a small portion of your time at the beginning of the week, you can enjoy the benefits for several days.

Consider prepping meals in advance or preparing frequently used ingredients in bulk. For instance, prepare a generous portion of your preferred protein sources. Simultaneously, cook a pot of nutritious brown rice and steam various vegetables like carrots, zucchini, and green beans. By doing so, you'll have a week's worth of ready-to-eat dinners conveniently stored in your fridge, awaiting your enjoyment.

Save time with frozen produce

When time is of the essence, it's best not to spend your limited time rinsing, peeling, and chopping vegetables. Instead, opt for the convenience of frozen vegetables. Ensure that the vegetable medleys you choose do not contain any high-FODMAP vegetables.

By stocking up on frozen vegetables, you can effortlessly enhance your savory meals with nutrient-dense options without spending extra time and money on fresh produce. This approach allows you to incorporate valuable vegetables into your diet while maintaining efficiency in your meal preparation.

Keep quick and easy options on hand

Stock your pantry with low-FODMAP convenience items like canned tuna, gluten-free pasta, rice cakes, low-FODMAP snack bars, and individually portioned servings of lactose-free yogurt or lactose-free milk.

General Baking Practices

When baking on a low FODMAP diet, there are some basic tips to keep in mind to ensure your creations are suitable for your dietary needs. Here are some baking tips for a low FODMAP diet:

- **Choose low FODMAP flour**: Choose gluten-free flours that are low in FODMAPs, such as rice flour, oat flour (certified gluten-free), tapioca flour, cornmeal, and almond flour. You can also find pre-made gluten-free flour blends suitable for a low FODMAP diet.

- **Replace high-FODMAP sweeteners**: Avoid high-FODMAP sweeteners like honey, agave syrup, and high-fructose corn syrup. Instead, choose low FODMAP options such as pure maple syrup, glucose syrup, or small amounts of table sugar (sucrose).

- **Use lactose-free dairy or alternatives**: If your recipe calls for dairy milk, use lactose-free milk or alternatives like almond or coconut milk. If butter is required, use lactose-free butter or a low-FODMAP oil (e.g., vegetable oil, coconut oil) as a substitute.

- **Choose low FODMAP flavorings:** Incorporate low FODMAP flavorings and extracts to add taste to your baked goods. Examples include pure vanilla extract, lemon zest, or low FODMAP spices and herbs like cinnamon, ginger, or nutmeg.

- **Be cautious with fruits:** While many fruits are high in FODMAPs, there are some low FODMAP options you can use in baking, such as berries (e.g., strawberries, blueberries, raspberries) and small portions of citrus fruits (e.g., lemon, lime). Keep the amount of fruit in your recipes within low FODMAP limits.

- **Substitute high FODMAP ingredients:** Look for suitable substitutions for high FODMAP ingredients in recipes. For instance, use Low Fodmap garlic-infused oil instead of whole garlic cloves, or replace onion with the green tops of spring onions (scallions) for a milder flavor.

How to eat out on a low FODMAP diet

Eating out while following a low FODMAP diet may initially seem challenging, but with some preparation and knowledge, it is possible to enjoy dining out without triggering digestive symptoms. Here are some tips to help you navigate eating out on a low-FODMAP diet:

- **Research the restaurant**: Before heading to a restaurant, do some research. Many restaurants now provide menus online so you can review them in advance. Look for dishes that are likely to be low FODMAP or can be easily modified. Call the restaurant beforehand to inquire about their ability to accommodate dietary restrictions.

- **Communicate your needs**: When you arrive at the restaurant, inform the waitstaff or server about your dietary requirements. Clearly explain that you are following a low FODMAP diet and need help selecting suitable options. Be polite but firm in conveying the importance of avoiding specific high FODMAP ingredients.

- **Focus on simple, unprocessed foods:** Opt for dishes that consist of simple, unprocessed ingredients. This gives you more control over what you're consuming and reduces the chances of consuming high FODMAP ingredients unknowingly.

- **Be cautious with sauces and dressings:** Many sauces, dressings, and condiments contain high FODMAP ingredients like onion, garlic, or honey. Ask for sauces and dressings to be served on the side, or request simple alternatives like olive oil, lemon juice, or vinegar.

- **Request modifications:** Don't hesitate to ask for modifications to suit your dietary needs. For example, ask for your burger without the bun or request that onion and garlic be omitted from a dish. Most restaurants are willing to accommodate dietary requests within reason.

- **Choose safe beverage options:** Be mindful of your beverage choices. Avoid high FODMAP drinks like fruit juices, sodas, or sweetened beverages. Choose water, herbal teas, or drinks you know are low FODMAP.

- **Be prepared with snacks**: If you're unsure about the available options or concerned about cross-contamination, carrying low-FODMAP snacks with you can be helpful. This ensures you have something to eat in case you cannot find suitable choices while dining out.

- **Practice portion control:** Remember that even low FODMAP foods can become problematic if consumed in large quantities. Practice portion control and listen to your body's signals of fullness.

- **Keep a food diary:** If you experience any digestive symptoms after eating out, it can be useful to maintain a food diary. Note down the specific foods you consumed and any symptoms that arise. This can help you identify potential trigger foods and make informed choices in the future.

Key Chapter Takeaways

- Reading food labels carefully is crucial when following a low-FODMAP diet to identify high-FODMAP ingredients or additives.

- Look for hidden sources of FODMAPs and be cautious of serving sizes and additive ingredients.

- Consider low-FODMAP certifications or labels on food products and be careful with "no added" claims.

- Keep a list of safe and trigger foods and consider cross-contamination in food processing.

- Stock your pantry with low FODMAP staples like not marinated meats, lactose-free dairy, gluten-free grains, specific vegetables and fruits, seasonings, low FODMAP bars, peanut butter, gluten-free all-purpose flour, pure maple syrup, salsa, and Low Fodmap garlic-infused olive oil.

- Keep your kitchen FODMAP friendly by stocking up on compliant starches, prepping food in advance, and rotating fruits and vegetables.

- Avoid high FODMAP foods such as garlic, onions, certain vegetables and fruits, beans and legumes, marinated or processed meats, certain dairy products, grains like barley, rye, and wheat, specific nuts and sweeteners, and certain beverages.

- Include low FODMAP foods like certain vegetables, fruits, meats, seafood, dairy alternatives, eggs, nuts and seeds, gluten-free bread and pasta, and specific sweeteners.

-Chapter 4-
7-Day Low Fodmap Meal Plan

Day 1:

Breakfast: Tortilla Baked Eggs

Preps In 5 Min, Cooks In 15 Min, Makes 1 Serving

Ingredients

- 1 tsp olive oil (for brushing the pan)
- 1 corn tortilla
- 1/2 cup baby kale or baby spinach (roughly chopped)
- eggs
- 1 tbsp green onions/scallions (green leaves only, finely chopped)
- cherry tomatoes (cut into quarters)
- 1/8 tsp paprika (small pinch)
- Season with salt & pepper
- 1 tbsp Colby or cheddar cheese or vegan cheese (optional) (grated)

Preparation

- Preheat the oven to 180°C/350°F.

- Roughly chop the spinach or kale. Finely slice the spring onion or green onion. Quarter the cherry tomatoes. Grate the cheese if you're using it.

- Grease a small oven-proof frypan or baking dish. Make sure the dish is slightly smaller than the tortilla. You can overlap the tortillas in a large dish or use multiple small baking dishes for multiple servings.

- Gently press the tortilla into the bottom of the dish, like with a pastry sheet. The edges of the tortilla should curl up slightly to form a lip that will hold the eggs.

- Evenly spread the spinach or kale over the tortilla.

- Crack the eggs on top, then sprinkle the spring onion, scallion leaves, and chopped tomato—season with a pinch of paprika, salt, and pepper. Add grated cheese if desired.

- Put the dish in the oven and bake for 15 to 20 minutes till the egg whites are set and no longer jiggly.

- Remove the low FODMAP tortilla-baked eggs from the oven and transfer them to a dish. Cut into quarters and enjoy!

Nutritional information

Calories: 402 | Fat: 24.5g | Protein: 25.6g | Carbs: 19.3g | Sugar: 4.5g

Low-FODMAP note:

- When choosing your tortilla wrap, be careful. Choose the one made from corn/maize flour that doesn't contain wheat flour or other high FODMAP ingredients.

- Check that the vegan cheese doesn't have onion, garlic, inulin, or coconut flour.

- When shopping, look out for spring onions or scallions with long green leaves. The white stem and lime green are high in FODMAP, but you can use the green leaves while on the low FODMAP diet.

Lunch: Asian Chicken Salad

Preps in 15 Min, Cooks in 15 Min, Makes 8 Servings

Ingredients

Peanut Butter Dressing:

- 6 tablespoons (102 g) peanut butter, either natural or no-stir style
- 3 tablespoons firmly packed light brown sugar
- 3 tablespoons of rice vinegar or apple cider vinegar
- 3 tablespoons low-sodium gluten-free soy sauce
- 11/2 tablespoons fish sauce
- 1 1/2 tablespoons of freshly squeezed lime juice
- 1 1/2 tablespoons Low Fodmap garlic-Infused Oil
- ¼ to ½ teaspoon sambal oelek or low FODMAP hot sauce
- Water, if needed

Chicken Salad:

- 1 red bell pepper, cored and finely sliced
- 1- pound (455 g) shredded cooked chicken warm or at room temperature
- 4 cups (356 g) finely shredded green cabbage
- 2 medium carrots, trimmed and grated

- 2 Persian cucumbers, ends trimmed, cut into large julienne
- 1/2 cup (16 g) of chopped fresh cilantro, divided
- 1/2 cup (80 g) chopped roasted peanuts, divided
- 1/2 cup (32 g) chopped scallions, green parts only, divided

Preparation

Peanut Butter Dressing:

- Combine peanut butter, brown sugar, vinegar, soy sauce, fish sauce, lime juice, oil, and hot sauce in a blender.

- Blend the ingredients till smooth and well combined, scraping down the sides of the blender as needed.

- Taste the dressing and add more hot sauce if desired. If using natural peanut butter and the mixture is too thick, blend in a tablespoon or two of water to achieve a smooth and pourable texture.

- For optimal flavor, the dressing can be made a day ahead and kept in an airtight container in the fridge.

Chicken Salad Assembly:

- Toss the chicken, cabbage, carrot, bell pepper, cucumbers, cilantro, half of the peanuts, and half of the scallions in a large mixing bowl.

- Add a portion of the dressing to the salad and gently toss to coat. Add enough dressing to coat the ingredients, as you may not need all the sauce.

- Serve the salad garnished with the remaining cilantro, peanuts, and scallions.

- The salad can be served with the chicken slightly warm or at room temperature.

Storage:

- The salad can be refrigerated in an airtight container for up to three days. Before serving, bring it to room temperature.

- For the best serving, garnish the salad with the remaining scallions, peanuts, and cilantro before serving.

- Alternatively, if you prefer to make the salad ahead of time, keep the salad and dressing separate until close to serving time. Add the garnishes just before serving for maximum freshness.

Nutritional information

Calories: 314 | Fat: 19g | Protein: 24g | Carbs: 15g | Sugar: 8g

Low-FODMAP note:

To make things easier, consider using a low FODMAP rotisserie chicken when preparing dishes that call for cooked chicken. Here's how to choose the right one:

- Look for rotisserie chicken labeled as "plain" or without added seasonings or sauces.

- Always read the labels to ensure there are no high FODMAP ingredients.

- It's also not a bad idea to check with your local supermarket to see if they offer low FODMAP rotisserie chickens.

Dinner: Whole Roast Chicken & Vegetables

Preps in 10 Min, Cooks in 1 Hr, Makes 6 Servings

Ingredients

- 3 tablespoons extra-virgin olive oil, divided
- 1.6 kg to 2 kg of whole chicken, giblets removed, patted dry
- 2 medium parsnips, scrubbed, trimmed, cut into 4-inch-long (10 cm) by ½-inch (12 mm) wide pieces
- 8- ounces (225 g) trimmed Brussels sprouts, halved lengthwise
- Freshly ground black pepper
- 4 medium carrots, scrubbed, trimmed, cut into 4-inch-long (10 cm) by ½-inch (12 mm) wide pieces
- Kosher salt

Procedure

- Pat the chicken dry with paper towels and generously season it with salt inside and out. Secure the legs with kitchen twine and allow the chicken to rest while the oven preheats.

- Position a rack in the upper third of the oven, ensuring enough space to accommodate the height of the chicken. Place a 12-inch to 14-inch (30.5 cm to 35.5 cm) cast-iron skillet in the oven and preheat it to 425°F (220°C).

- In the meantime, toss the carrots, parsnips, and Brussels sprouts with half of the olive oil in a large bowl, ensuring all the vegetables are seasoned with salt and pepper to taste.

- Coat the chicken with some reserved oil once the oven reaches the desired temperature. Drizzle the left-over oil into the hot skillet. Carefully place the chicken in the center of the skillet and scatter the vegetables around it. Roast in the oven for approximately 50 to 60 minutes. Allow the chicken to cool in the skillet for at least 10 minutes.

- Move the chicken to a cutting board and carve it. Serve the succulent chicken alongside the roasted vegetables.

Nutritional information

Calories: 300 | Fat: 14g | Protein: 29g | Carbs: 13g | Sugar: 4g

Day 2:

Breakfast: Berry Nice Muesli

Preps In 10 Min, Cooks In 25 Min, Makes 10 Servings

Ingredients

- 300 g (3 cups) rolled oats
- 80 g (1 cup) dried shredded coconut
- 115 g (1 cup) pecan (chopped)
- 105 g (3/4 cup) pumpkin seeds
- 4 tbsp   pure maple syrup
- 4 tbsp   olive oil
- 2 tbsp   brown sugar
- 1 1/2 tsp   vanilla extract
- 8 tbsp   dried cranberries
- 12 g (1 cup) freeze-dried strawberries (chopped)

Procedure

- Heat the oven to 160°C/320°F and line a deep roasting tray with baking paper.

- Mix the maple syrup, olive oil, brown sugar, and vanilla in a small bowl.

- Combine the oats, coconut, chopped pecans, and pumpkin seeds in a bowl. Pour in the sugar mixture and mix everything.

- Pour the oat mixture into the prepared roasting tray, spreading it evenly in a shallow layer. Put the tray in the middle of the oven and bake for 20 minutes. Then, stir it and continue baking for another 10 to 15 minutes till it turns golden.

- Remove the tray from the oven and carefully mix in the dried cranberries and strawberries.

- Allow the mixture to cool, then move it to an airtight container. It can be stored for up to three weeks.

- When ready to enjoy, serve ¾ cup portions with your choice of low-FODMAP milk and yogurt.

Nutritional information

Calories: 423 | Fat: 26.3g | Protein: 8.8g | Carbs: 42.4g | Sugar: 16.8g

Low-FODMAP note:

- Ensure to use pure maple syrup (low FODMAP) and not maple-flavored syrup (high FODMAP)

- Ensure the dried cranberries are not sweetened with apple juice but with sugar.

Lunch: Macaroni Slaw

Preps in 15 Min, Cooks in 15 Min, Makes 14 Servings

Ingredients

- 12 ounces (340 g) low FODMAP gluten-free elbow pasta, cooked al dente, drained, and cooled
- 1/4 cup (60 g) lactose-free sour cream
- 1 cup (226 g) of mayonnaise
- 8 ounces (225 g) green cabbage, shredded
- 1 tablespoon sugar
- 1 medium green bell pepper, cored and diced
- 8 ounces (225 g) of red cabbage, shredded
- 2 medium carrots, scrubbed, root end trimmed, shredded
- 2 medium stalks of celery, diced
- 1/4 cup (16 g) finely chopped scallions, green parts only
- 1 teaspoon celery seeds
- 1/4 cup (60 ml) of apple cider vinegar
- Kosher salt
- Freshly ground black pepper

Preparation

- Combine the drained and cooled pasta, red and green cabbage, shredded carrot, diced celery, bell pepper, and chopped scallions in a mixing bowl.

- Whisk together the mayo, vinegar, sour cream, sugar, and celery seed in a small mixing bowl. Taste the dressing and adjust the seasoning with salt and pepper according to your preference.

- Pour the dressing directly over the pasta and vegetables, and gently fold everything until well mixed.

- The salad is ready to be served, but let it sit for at least 1 hour for the best flavor to allow the flavors to meld together. Alternatively, you can refrigerate the salad overnight in an airtight container.

- Before serving, let the salad cool to room temperature or serve it lightly chilled for optimal enjoyment.

- The salad can be stored in the fridge for up to three days in an airtight container.

Nutritional information

Calories: 227 | Fat: 14g | Protein: 3g | Carbs: 22g | Sugar: 2g

Dinner: *Chicken & Sausage Jambalaya*

Preps in 10 Min, Cooks in 50 Min, Makes 6 Servings

Ingredients

- 6 medium chicken thighs, skin on, bone in
- 2 teaspoons paprika
- 2 teaspoons kosher salt
- 1 teaspoon black pepper
- 1 teaspoon oregano
- 1 teaspoon thyme
- ¼ to 1 teaspoon chipotle chile powder
- 4 cups (960 ml) water
- 1, 28 ounce (793 g) can of diced tomatoes, preferably fire-roasted
- 1 pound (455 g) low FODMAP sausage (we used a sweet sausage)
- 1/4 cup (60 ml) Low Fodmap garlic-Infused Oil
- 1 medium green bell pepper cored, seeded, and diced
- 1/2 cup (36 g) chopped leeks, green parts only
- 1/2 cup (32 g) chopped scallions, green parts only
- 1 medium celery stalk, diced
- 1 bay leaf
- 2 cups (370 g) long-grain white rice

Preparation

- Mix the chicken thighs with paprika, salt, pepper, oregano, thyme, and chipotle chile in a mixing bowl. Toss the chicken thighs in the spice mixture until they are well coated. Set it aside.

- Bring water or stock to a boil over medium heat in a medium-sized saucepan. Prick the sausages in a few places and add them to the boiling liquid. Simmer for about 5 minutes or until the sausages are halfway cooked. Remove the sausages from the liquid and set them aside on a cutting board to cool. Save the cooking water for later use. Cut the sausages into 1-inch (2.5 cm) pieces.

- In a skillet, heat oil over medium heat. Add the chicken thighs, skin side down, and brown them for about 5 minutes until nicely browned. Flip the chicken over and brown the other side as well. The chicken should be about three-quarters cooked through. Remove the chicken from the pan.

- Add the leek, scallion greens, bell pepper, and celery to the same skillet. Sauté the vegetables for about 3 minutes, stirring often, until softened but not browned. Stir in the tomatoes and bay leaf, and then add the rice and 4 cups (960 ml) of the reserved sausage cooking water/stock. Top off with water to reach 4 cups (960 ml) if needed. Nestle the chicken pieces in the sauce, skin side up, and scatter the sausage pieces around them. Cover the skillet, boil the mixture, then reduce the heat and cook for 20 to 30 mins until the rice is cooked and most liquid is absorbed. The jambalaya should have a juicy consistency. The Chicken & Sausage Jambalaya is now ready to be served. It can also be refrigerated in an airtight container for up to 3 days and reheated gently on the stovetop or microwave.

Nutritional information

- Calories: 756 | Fat: 47g | Protein: 30g | Carbs: 72g | Sugar: 4g

Day 3:

Breakfast: Quinoa Porridge with Berries and Cinnamon

Preps In 2 Min, Cooks In 25 Min, Makes 2 Servings

Ingredients

- 85 g (1/2 cup) quinoa
- 1 tsp neutral oil (rice bran, canola, sunflower)
- 250 ml (1 cup) water
- 188 ml (3/4 cup) low FODMAP milk
- 1/4 tsp ground cinnamon
- 4 tsp pure maple syrup
- 10 raspberries (fresh or frozen)
- 20 blueberries (fresh or frozen)

Procedure

- Measure the quinoa and rinse it under cold running water for two minutes using a fine mesh sieve. Transfer the rinsed quinoa to a medium-sized saucepan and add a drizzle of neutral oil.

- Toast the quinoa overheat for 1 to 2 minutes until the water evaporates and the quinoa is lightly toasted.

- Add the water to the saucepan. Bring the quinoa to a rolling boil, then reduce the heat to the lowest setting. Cover the pan with a lid and allow the quinoa to cook for 12 to 15 minutes until it becomes fluffy.

- If there is excess water, drain it and return the quinoa to the pan.

- Add the low-FODMAP milk, cinnamon, and maple syrup to the pan. If the low FODMAP milk is absorbed completely, you can add more if desired. Allow the porridge to cook for about 5 minutes or till heated through. If you're using frozen berries and want them heated, add them to the mixture.

- Serve the hot quinoa porridge in bowls and evenly divide the raspberries and blueberries between them.

Nutritional information

Calories: 251 | Fat: 6.2g | Protein: 6.8g | Carbs: 42.8g | Sugar: 11.5g

Low-FODMAP note:

- Ensure to use pure maple syrup (low FODMAP) and not maple-flavored syrup (high FODMAP)

- Lactose-free milk, almond milk, hemp milk, macadamia milk, quinoa milk, rice milk, and soy milk made from soy protein (not whole or hulled soybeans) are examples of low FODMAP milk.

- Ensure the low-FODMAP milk doesn't contain ingredients like inulin (chicory root), agave syrup, fructose, high fructose corn syrup, molasses, or honey.

Lunch: Vegan Chickpea Salad

Preps in 10 Min, Cooks in 10 Min, Makes 8 Servings

Ingredients

- 1, 15.5- ounce (439 g) chickpeas, drained, rinsed, and drained
- 1 teaspoon of Dijon mustard
- 1 medium carrot, trimmed and chopped
- ¼ teaspoon of dried dill
- 2 tablespoons finely chopped flat leaf parsley: optional
- ¼ cup (16 g) of finely chopped scallions, green parts only
- ¼ cup (56 g) vegan mayonnaise
- 1 teaspoon lemon juice
- 1 Persian cucumber, trimmed and chopped
- Kosher salt
- Freshly ground black pepper

Preparation

- Put the drained chickpeas in a mixing bowl and use a fork or pastry blender to mash them, creating a chunky texture partially.

- Add the shredded carrot, diced cucumber, sliced scallions, and chopped parsley (if desired) to the bowl. Mix them with the mashed chickpeas.

- Fold in the mayo, mustard, lemon juice, and dill, ensuring all the ingredients are well combined.

- Taste the chickpea salad and season it with salt and pepper according to your preference.

- The chickpea salad is now ready to be enjoyed! Alternatively, you can refrigerate it in an airtight container for up to 3 days.

- Serve the chickpea salad on a plate, use it as a sandwich filling, pair it with low-FODMAP crackers or pretzels, or simply enjoy it with a spoon!

Nutritional information

Calories: 122 | Fat: 6g | Protein: 3g | Carbs: 15g | Sugar: 1g

Low-FODMAP note:

For a delightful low FODMAP Chickpea Salad Stuffed Tomato:

- Select firm beefsteak tomatoes, allowing one tomato per serving. Cut about ¼-inch off the stem end, creating a flat surface.

- Use a spoon to carefully scoop out the middle of the tomato, creating a hollow bowl-like shape.

- Fill the tomato bowl with your delicious chickpea salad, packing it gently for a satisfying filling.

- To add a decorative touch, create little jagged edges on the tomato using a sharp paring knife if desired. Make one cut at a time, creating a visually appealing presentation.

Dinner: Oven-baked egg & chips

Preps in 5 Min, Cooks in 35 Min, Makes 2 Servings

Ingredients

- 2 medium baking potatoes, cut into chunky wedges
- 2 tbsp olive oil
- 1 tsp smoked paprika
- 2 tomatoes, halved
- 2 eggs

Preparation

- Heat the oven to 190°C.

- Place the potato wedges in a roasting tin. Drizzle them with oil and sprinkle paprika over them. Season with salt and pepper and mix well to ensure the potatoes are evenly coated.

- Roast in the oven for 25 mins, tossing them halfway through until they are almost tender.

- Gently nestle the tomatoes, cut side up, among the potatoes. Create two spaces in the tin and carefully crack an egg into each space.

- Return the tin to the oven and bake for 6-8 minutes or until the eggs are set.

Nutritional information

Calories: 327 | Fat: 19g | Protein: 11g | Carbs: 25g | Sugar: 3g

Day 4

Breakfast: Mini Banana Pancakes

Prep In 5 Min, Cooks In 20 Min, Makes 2 Servings (4 Mini Pancakes Per Serving)

Ingredients

- 160 g (2 small) bananas (firm - no brown spots)
- 2 large eggs
- 2 tbsp gluten-free all-purpose flour
- 1 tbsp brown sugar
- 1/4 tsp baking powder
- 1/8 tsp salt (a good pinch)
- 1/2 tsp ground cinnamon
- 1/4 tsp ground nutmeg
- 3 tbsp butter or dairy-free spread (for cooking)

Procedure

- In a large bowl, peel the bananas and mash them until smooth. Whisk in the eggs until well combined.

- Add the baking powder, salt, gluten-free flour, cinnamon, nutmeg, and brown sugar to the bowl. Mix everything until well combined.

- Heat a frying pan over medium heat. Add a tablespoon of dairy-free spread or butter to the pan.

- Scoop about 3 tablespoons of batter for each pancake into the pan. Allow the batter to cook until small bubbles start forming on top. Check the underside of the pancake, and gently flip it if it's golden brown. Cook each pancake until both sides are golden brown. Add more dairy-free spread to the pan as needed. If the pan becomes too hot, reduce to a medium-low temperature.

- Serve the pancakes by layering them with low-FODMAP yogurt and blueberries.

- If desired, dust the pancakes with powdered sugar/icing sugar for an extra touch.

Nutritional information

Calories: 479 | Fat: 33.1g | Protein: 10.5g | Carbs: 36.5g | Sugar: 19.6g

Low-FODMAP note:

- Before buying coconut yoghurt or lactose-free yoghurt, check the label for inulin (chicory root) and high FODMAP sweeteners such as honey, agave syrup, fructose, fruit juice, high fructose corn syrup, or high FODMAP fruits. Avoid products that contain these ingredients to ensure they are low in FODMAP.

- When selecting bananas, opt for common bananas rather than sugar bananas. Use bananas when they are firm, ranging from green to just yellow. Ripe bananas with brown spots are considered high FODMAP.

- Choose gluten-free plain flour or gluten-free all-purpose flour. Ensure that the flour blends you select do not contain soy flour, chickpea/besan/gram/garbanzo bean flour, lentil flour, coconut flour, amaranth flour, or lupin flour. Look for a blend that includes maize starch, rice flour, tapioca starch, rice bran, and guar gum.

Lunch: Warm Bacon & Avocado Salad

Preps in 10 Min, Cooks in 10 Min, Makes 8 Servings

Ingredients

Salad:

- Selection of lettuces and salad greens, such as butterhead, iceberg, Belgian endive, radicchio, trevisano, watercress, and salad burnet
- 6- ounces (170 g) slab bacon, unsmoked or lightly smoked
- Clarified butter, or a mixture of butter and oil, plus olive oil, for cooking the bacon
- 4 slices low FODMAP white bread
- Sunflower or olive oil for cooking the croutons
- 1 avocado (160 g total)
- 18 fresh walnut halves to garnish (optional)

Dressing:

- 3 tablespoons walnut oil or a mixture of 2 tablespoons walnut oil and 1 tablespoon sunflower oil
- 1 tablespoon Chardonnay wine vinegar
- 1 teaspoon freshly chopped chives
- 1 teaspoon freshly chopped flat-leaf parsley
- Sea salt and freshly ground black pepper

Preparation

Prepare the Salad:

- Begin by thoroughly washing and drying the salad greens. Tear them into bite-size pieces and place them in a bowl. Cover the bowl and refrigerate till ready to use.

Making the Croutons:

- Remove the rind from the bacon and cut it into ¼-inch (6 mm) cubes. In a skillet, cook the bacon in a combination of clarified butter or a mixture of butter and oil until it turns golden. Once cooked, drain the bacon on paper towels.

- For the croutons, start by cutting off the crusts from the bread. Then, slice the bread into strips about ¼ inch (6 mm) wide and dice them into precise cubes. Heat at least ¾ inch (2 cm) of sunflower or olive oil in a skillet until it is almost smoking. Carefully add the bread cubes to the hot oil and stir gently. The croutons will quickly become golden brown. Place a strainer over a Pyrex or stainless-steel bowl and pour the oil and croutons into the strainer. Let the excess oil drain, and then transfer the croutons to paper towels. You can prepare the croutons several hours or even a day in advance.

Making the Dressing:

- In a bowl, whisk the liquid ingredients for the dressing until well combined. Add the chopped herbs and season with salt and freshly ground pepper to taste.

- Halve the avocado and remove the pit. Peel it and dice the flesh into ½-inch (12 mm) pieces.

Serve:

- Toss the salad greens with just enough dressing to give them a light, glistening coating. Add the warm, crispy croutons and diced avocado. Gently toss the salad to combine all the ingredients. Divide the salad evenly among eight plates.

- In a hot skillet, reheat the bacon with a splash of olive oil until it becomes crisp and golden. Scatter the hot bacon over the salad for added flavor and texture.

- For an optional garnish, you can include walnut halves. Serve the salad immediately, allowing the delightful combination of flavors and textures to be enjoyed at its best.

Nutritional information

Calories: 246 | Fat: 1g | Protein: 5g | Carbs: 9g | Sugar: 1g

Dinner: Stir Fry

Preps in 10 Min, Cooks in 10 Min, Makes 1 Servings

Ingredients

- 1 Tbsp olive oil Low Fodmap garlic-infused
- 1/2 to 1 cup mixed vegetables steamer bags
- 1/2 cup chicken
- 1/2 to 1 cup cooked rice
- soy sauce low sodium

Preparation

- Heat the Low Fodmap garlic-infused oil over medium-high heat in a wok or large saucepan.

- Prepare the vegetables by cutting them into small pieces. Add them to the wok and begin stirring.

- Take the chicken and cut it into bite-sized pieces. Season with salt and pepper.

- Once the vegetables have started to soften, add the seasoned chicken to the hot wok. Stir constantly for 2 to 3 minutes.

- Continue stirring until the chicken and vegetables are fully cooked and nicely browned. You can add the rice to the pan for the last few minutes of cooking or serve it on the side.

- When everything is cooked to your desired level, pour in the sauce and sauté for a few more minutes, allowing the flavors to meld together.

Nutritional information

Calories: 514 | Fat: 26g | Protein: 19g | Carbs: 51g

Day 5

Breakfast: Egg Shakshuka

Preps In 5 Min, Cooks In 20 Min, Makes 4 Servings

Ingredients

- green bell pepper (deseeded & cut into strips)
- 60 g (2 cups) baby spinach (roughly chopped)
- 10 g (1/4 cup) green onions/scallions (green tips only, finely chopped)
- 1 tbsp Low Fodmap garlic-infused oil
- 400 g plain tomatoes canned
- 250 ml (1 cup) low FODMAP chicken stock/vegetable stock
- 1 tbsp cornstarch
- 1 tsp paprika
- 1 tsp ground cumin
- 1/8 tsp dried chili flakes
- 1/2 tsp white sugar
- Season with salt & pepper
- 4 large eggs
- 8 slices low FODMAP bread (for serving)

Procedure

- Begin by deseeding and chopping the green pepper/capsicum into thick strips. Chop the spinach, and finely chop the green onions/scallions (using only the green tips).

- Heat a large frypan over medium-high heat. Add the Low Fodmap garlic-infused oil and the chopped pepper/capsicum. Fry them until they start to soften.

- Add the tomatoes and chicken stock to the pan. Mix well and let the sauce simmer for two minutes.

- In a small amount of warm water, dissolve the cornstarch and stir it into the sauce. Add most of the spinach (reserving some for garnish) and the chopped green onions/scallions (green tips only). Allow the sauce to cook for two more minutes till it thickens.

- Stir in the paprika, cumin, chili flakes, and sugar—season with salt and pepper. Taste the sauce and add more seasoning and spices (like chili flakes) to meet your desired level of spiciness. Reduce the heat to medium-low.

- Break the eggs into the tomato mixture, spacing them around the frypan. Cover the frypan with a lid and let it simmer for 10 to 15 minutes or until the eggs are cooked to your liking.

- Sprinkle the remaining spinach over the dish for garnish. Serve the shakshuka with a side of toasted low-FODMAP bread.

Nutritional information

Calories: 346 | Fat: 11.7g | Protein: 17.3g | Carbs: 45.1g | Sugar: 9.3g

Low-FODMAP note:

- When buying, look out for spring onions or scallions with long green leaves. The white stem and lime green are high in FODMAP, but you can use the green leaves in low FOD-MAP.

- Ensure that the corn flour (corn starch) you use is made from maize and contains no wheat.

- Check your dried chili flakes to ensure they do not contain onion or garlic powder as ingredients.

- When selecting canned tomatoes, choose plain ones without any added herbs, spices, onion, or garlic.

- Avoid ingredients such as inulin, apple or pear juice, apple fiber, concentrated fruit juices, honey, or high fructose corn syrup to ensure a low FODMAP recipe.

- Additionally, be mindful of the type of flour used in your recipes. Avoid products that contain amaranth flour, chickpea, besa, gram, garbanzo bean flour, lentil flour, lupin flour, soy flour or coconut flour.

Lunch: Baked Sea Bass with lemon caper dressing

Preps in 10 Min, Cooks in 10 Min, Makes 4 Servings

Ingredients

- Olive oil for brushing
- 4 x 100g/4oz of sea bass fillets

For the caper dressing:

- 3 tbsp of extra virgin olive oil
- 2 tsp of gluten-free Dijon mustard
- 2 tbsp of chopped flat-leaf parsley, plus a few extra leaves (optional)
- 2 tbsp small capers
- Grated zest 1 lemon, plus 2 tbsp of juice

Preparation

Prepare the Dressing

- Combine the oil, lemon zest, lemon juice, capers, mustard, and a pinch of seasoning in a bowl. However, hold off on adding the parsley until you plan to serve the dish immediately. Mixing the parsley too early can cause its color to fade due to the acid in the lemon. If you're not serving the dish immediately, reserve the parsley to add later.

Cooking the Fish

- Preheat your oven to 220C.
- Line a baking tray with baking parchment.

- Put the fish fillets on the prepared baking tray, skin-side up. Brush the skin with a thin layer of oil and sprinkle some flaky salt over it to enhance the flavor and texture.

- Bake the fish in the heated oven for approximately 7 minutes or until the flesh easily flakes when tested with a knife. Cooking times may vary on the thickness of the fillets.

Serve:

- Gently transfer the cooked fish to warm serving plates. Spoon the prepared dressing over the fish, generously coating each fillet with its vibrant flavors.

- If desired, sprinkle additional parsley leaves over the dressed fish to add a touch of freshness and visual appeal.

Nutritional information

Calories: 205 | Fat: 13g | Protein: 20g | Carbs: 1g | Sugar: 1g

Dinner: Thai Pumpkin Noodle Soup

Preps In 10 Min, Cooks In 55 Min, Makes 6 Servings

Ingredients

Roasted Vegetables

- 850 g   Japanese pumpkin (Kabocha squash or Buttercup squash) (peeled, deseeded & cut into cubes)
- 250 g   carrots (peeled & cut into cubes)
- 1 tsp   ground cumin
- Drizzle of olive oil
- Season with   salt & pepper

Other Soup Ingredients

- 500 ml (2 cups) low FODMAP chicken stock/vegetable stock
- 40 g (1 cup) green onions/scallions (green tips only, finely chopped)
- 1 tsp   crushed ginger
- 1/2 tsp   lemon zest
- 2 tsp   Thai fish sauce (nam pla) or soy sauce
- 1/8 tsp   dried chili flakes (start with a pinch and add more to taste)
- 375 ml (1 1/2 cup) coconut milk (canned)
- 250 g   thin rice noodles
- 1/4 cup   fresh cilantro (chopped)

Preparation

- Heat your oven to 180°C/350°F using the bake function.

- Remove the seeds and skin from the pumpkin, then cut it into 3cm (1.2 inch) cubes. Cube the carrot as well. Place both vegetables in a roasting tray and drizzle with oil, ensuring they are well coated. Sprinkle with cumin, salt, and pepper for added flavor. Bake in the oven for 20 to 30 mins, turning once, until they become soft and golden (be careful not to burn them).

- Allow the roasted veggies to cool for about 10 minutes, then blend them with the stock until smooth.

- Heat a large saucepan over medium heat. Drizzle a small amount of olive oil into the pan and sauté the spring onion tips for 2 to 3 minutes until they become fragrant. Next, add the ginger and continue cooking for an additional minute.

- Introduce the pureed pumpkin and coconut milk to the saucepan, stirring well to combine. Incorporate the vibrant flavors of lemon zest, fish sauce (or soy sauce), and chili flakes into the mixture. Allow the soup to simmer gently over low heat for 10 to 15 minutes.

- If the soup has thickened too much, simply add a splash of boiling water to achieve your desired consistency and texture. This will help to maintain a smooth and velvety consistency throughout the soup.

- While the soup simmers, cook the noodles according to the instructions on the packet. To prevent them from getting soggy, slightly undercook them for 1 to 2 minutes.

- Stir the cooked noodles into the soup and the fresh coriander/cilantro. Serve immediately and enjoy your flavorful pumpkin and vegetable noodle soup!

Nutritional information

Calories: 373 | Fat: 16.3g | Protein: 7.4g | Carbs: 52.6g | Sugar: 8.1g

Day 6

Breakfast: Sweet Potato Hash

Preps In 5 Min, Cooks In 20 Min, Makes 4 Servings

Ingredients

- 2 large, sweet potato
- 6 tbsp vegetable oil
- 1 bell pepper chopped
- 1 lb ground turkey
- 1/2 cup scallion (green part), chopped
- salt
- black pepper
- 2 tbsp fresh parsley

Procedure

- Cook two sweet potatoes in the microwave until tender but not mushy. Peel them and cut them into small cubes.

- In a skillet, heat two tablespoons of oil over medium-high heat. Add the bell pepper and cook till it becomes tender. Then, add the ground turkey, breaking it up as it cooks. Once the turkey is cooked, add the green part of the scallions and cook for another minute. Transfer the mixture to a bowl and set it aside.

- In the same skillet, add the remaining four tablespoons of oil. Place the sweet potato cubes in a single layer and let them cook undisturbed for about five minutes until they turn golden brown. Stir them gently and allow them to continue cooking until all the potatoes are golden.

- Return the turkey mixture to the skillet with the sweet potatoes. Season everything generously with salt and pepper.

- Top the dish with parsley for added freshness and flavor.

- Enjoy your delicious meal!

Nutrition information

Calories: 475 | Fat: 23g | Protein: 30g | Carbs: 37g

Lunch: Salmon Sushi Bowl

Preps In 5 Min, Cooks In 20 Min, Makes 2 Servings

Ingredients

SUSHI RICE

- 105 g (1/2 cup) short-grain sushi rice (uncooked)
- 4 tsp   rice wine vinegar
- 1 1/2 tsp   white sugar

GLAZED SALMON

- 300 g   fresh salmon fillets (bones removed)
- 2 tsp Low Fodmap garlic-infused oil
- 1 tbsp   soy sauce
- 1/4 tsp   crushed ginger
- 2 tsp   brown sugar
- 1/2 tsp   rice wine vinegar
- 1/2 tsp   sesame oil

OTHER INGREDIENTS

- small cucumber
- 4   radishes
- 60 g (4 tbsp) avocados
- nori seaweed sheet (optional)
- 1/2 tsp   sesame seeds (light sprinkle)
- 2 tsp   green onions/scallions (green leaves only, finely chopped)

LIME MAYONNAISE

- 3 tbsp mayonnaise
- Large lime (use 1/2 of the zest and juice of a lime for every 2 serves)

Preparation

- Heat the oven to 200°C/390°F.

- Cook the sushi rice using the absorption method indicated in the packet instructions.

- Line a roasting pan with baking paper for easy cleanup.

Soy Glazed Salmon:

- Combine the Low Fodmap garlic oil, soy sauce, ginger, vinegar, brown sugar, and sesame oil in a bowl to create a flavorful glaze.

- Place the salmon fillets in the roasting pan, skin side down, and brush them with half of the soy glaze mixture.

- Bake the salmon in the heated oven for 6 minutes, then brush with more soy glaze and bake for an additional 6 minutes until cooked through.

- For an irresistible caramelized finish, briefly grill/broil the salmon in the oven for 1 to 2 minutes.

- Remove the salmon from the oven and set it aside while you prepare the remaining components.

Lime Mayo and Vegetable Preparation:

- Mix the mayo, lime zest, and lime juice in a separate bowl until well combined to create a zesty lime mayo.

- Peel and slice the cucumber into chunky shapes, thinly slice the radish, and measure out the avocado.

- Cut the nori into small strips using scissors for added texture and flavor.

Sushi Rice and Assembly:

- Once the sushi rice is cooked, fluff it with a fork and mix in the rice wine vinegar and white sugar. Adjust the sweetness to your liking.

- Divide the cooked sushi rice, glazed salmon, and prepared vegetables into individual serving bowls.

- Garnish each bowl with nori strips, sesame seeds, and finely sliced spring onion/scallion leaves for an appealing presentation.

- Drizzle a generous amount of lime mayo over the ingredients for a tangy finish.

- Serve the dish with extra slices of lime on the side, allowing each person to customize their flavors.

Nutritional information

Calories: 606 | Fat: 22.6g | Protein: 37.6g | Carbs: 62.6g | Sugar: 10.6g

Low-FODMAP note:

- When buying Low Fodmap garlic-infused oil, ensure it is clear without any garlic bits.

- Check that crushed ginger does not contain garlic or use fresh ginger as a substitute. Nori sheets can be found in Asian food stores or supermarkets.

- When buying spring onions/scallions, opt for those with long green leaves, avoiding the white and light green stems.

- Avocado is low FODMAP in small amounts. Stick to a serving size of 2 tablespoons (30g/1.06oz).

- Regular soy sauce typically contains low wheat, but gluten-free soy sauce is available if needed.

- Select a mayonnaise that does not contain onion or garlic powder for a low FODMAP option.

Dinner: Potato & Egg Salad

Preps In 5 Min, Cooks In 25 Min, Makes 4 Servings

Ingredients

- 800 g potatoes
- 160 g green beans
- 4 large eggs
- 0.75 red bell pepper
- small cucumber
- 3 tbsp fresh chives
- 3 tbsp green onions/scallions (green tips only)
- 85 ml (1/3 cup) mayonnaise
- 1 tbsp lemon juice
- 1 tbsp wholegrain mustard
- Season with black pepper

Preparation

- Begin by scrubbing the potatoes thoroughly and cutting them into bite-sized pieces. If necessary, peel the potatoes before cutting. Similarly, trim the ends of the green beans and cut them into small pieces.

- Take a large saucepan and add the potato pieces to it. Cover the potatoes with water, place the lid on the saucepan, and set it over medium-high heat. Bring the water to a rolling boil. Once boiling, reduce the heat to medium-low. Let the potatoes simmer for 15 to 20 minutes until they become tender. Add the green beans to the saucepan for approximately 3 minutes before draining the potatoes. Cook them for an extra 2 to 3 minutes until they are tender yet still vibrant. Drain the vegetables and put them aside to cool.

- While the potatoes are cooking, prepare the hard-boiled eggs. Put the eggs in a saucepan and cover them with cold water. Bring the water to a rolling boil over medium-high heat and let it boil for two minutes. Reduce the heat to the lowest and cook the eggs for 10 to 12 minutes. Once done, drain the eggs and rinse them under cold water to cool them down. Peel the eggs and cut them into quarters.

- While the eggs cook, prepare the cucumber and red bell peppers. Peel the cucumber and cut it into short sticks. Remove the seeds from the red bell peppers and dice them into small pieces. Finely chop the green onion, using only the green tips and the chives.

- Whisk the mayonnaise, wholegrain mustard, lemon juice, and a few black pepper grinds in a different bowl. This will create a flavorful and creamy salad dressing.

- In a large bowl, gently mix the cooked potatoes, green beans, hard-boiled eggs, cucumber, red bell peppers, green onions, chives, and salad dressing. Season the salad with a few more grinds of black pepper.

- Enjoy.

Nutritional information

Calories: 324 | Fat: 11.2g | Protein: 13.4g | Carbs: 43.7g | Sugar: 5.9g

Day 7

Breakfast: Breakfast Buckwheat

Preps In 5 Min, Cooks In 10 Min, Makes 3 Servings

Ingredients

- 2 of cups water
- 1 cup of buckwheat groats
- 1/4 of tsp salt
- 1/2 of tsp cinnamon
- 1 tsp of vanilla extract
- 1/4 of cup almond milk or desired milk alternative

Procedure

- In a saucepan, combine water and groats.

- Stir in salt, cinnamon, and vanilla to enhance the flavors.

- Bring the mixture to a boil, cover the saucepan, and reduce the heat to a simmer. Let it simmer for 10 minutes, allowing the groats to absorb the liquid and soften.

- Stir in milk to add creaminess to the dish. Continue to cook, stirring occasionally, until you achieve your desired consistency.

- Remove the saucepan from the heat once the groats reach the desired consistency.

- Serve the groats in bowls and garnish them with your favorite toppings.

Nutrition information

Calories: 221 | Fat: 2g | Protein: 8g | Carbs: 41g | Sugar: 3g

Lunch: Creamy Ham and Potato Soup

Preps In 10 Min, Cooks In 30 Min, Makes 4 Servings

Ingredients

- 195 g (1 1/2 cup) shaved ham (we used leftover Christmas ham)
- 80 g (1 cup) leek (green leaves only, finely chopped)
- 800 g potatoes (peeled & chopped in small chunks)
- 240 g (2 large) carrots (peeled & diced)
- 2 tbsp butter or dairy-free spread
- 1 tbsp Low Fodmap garlic-infused oil
- 2 tbsp gluten-free all-purpose flour
- 625 ml (2 1/2 cups) low FODMAP chicken stock
- 375 ml (1 1/2 cup) low FODMAP milk
- 6 tbsp sweet corn kernels (frozen or fresh)
- 1 tsp dried chives
- Season with salt & pepper
- 2 tsp fresh parsley (finely chopped, optional)

Preparation

- Prepare the ham, leek leaves, potato, and carrot, and measure the sweet corn.

- Melt the dairy-free spread or butter in a large saucepan over medium heat. Sauté the leek leaves and carrot for 3 minutes until the carrot softens.

- Next, add the potato, ham, and Low Fodmap garlic-infused oil. Cook for 2 minutes, stirring sporadically to prevent the vegetables from sticking.

- Incorporate the flour into the mixture and cook for an additional minute. Then pour in the stock, stirring well, and bring to a boil. Allow it to simmer for 12 minutes, stirring occasionally, till the potatoes are soft.

- Reduce the heat to medium-low and add the sweet corn, milk, and dried chives. Stir the soup over the heat until it thickens, approximately 5 mins.

- Taste the soup and season with salt and pepper if necessary.

- Serve the soup warm and optionally garnish with a sprinkle of parsley.

- If the soup becomes too thick, simply stir in a splash of milk to adjust the consistency.

Nutritional information

Calories: 424 | Fat: 15.7g | Protein: 16.6g | Carbs: 57.5g | Sugar: 8.1g

Low-FODMAP note:

- Ensure that the shaved ham you choose does not contain high fructose corn syrup as a curing ingredient. Ham cured with honey is a suitable option since honey has a small low

FODMAP serving size, and the amount used in one serving of ham should comply with low FODMAP guidelines.

- When selecting a stock, choose a variety that does not contain onion or garlic.

Dinner: Tasty Salmon Fritters

Preps In 5 Min, Cooks In 10 Min, Makes 2 Servings

Ingredients

Fritters

- 210 g   plain pink salmon (canned)
- 20 g (1/4 cup) green leek tips or spring onion tips (sliced)
- large egg (lightly beaten)
- 1 tsp   crushed ginger*
- 1 tsp   sesame oil
- Season with   salt & pepper
- 2 tbsp   mayonnaise (to serve)

Vermicelli Noodle Serving Suggestion

- 170 g   bok choy (pak choi)
- 50 g   rice vermicelli noodles (dry weight)

Burger Serving Suggestion

- 2   gluten free burger buns
- 70 g (2 cups) lettuce (butter, iceberg, red coral) (to serve)
- medium common tomato

Procedure

- Begin by opening and draining the can of salmon. Transfer the salmon to a medium-sized bowl. Finely slice the green leek tips or spring onion tips. Lightly beat the egg and add it to the bowl with sliced green leek tips, crushed ginger, toasted sesame oil, and a pinch of salt and pepper. Thoroughly mix the ingredients until well combined. The mixture will have a chunky and moist consistency.

- Heat a large frying pan and coat it with non-stick oil spray or a thin layer of olive oil applied with a paper towel. Spoon 1/4 cup portions of the salmon mixture directly onto the pan, allowing space for 4 patties per batch. Cook the patties for 4 minutes on each side until they turn golden brown. Be patient and avoid flipping them too early to prevent them from falling apart.

- For the rice vermicelli option, stir-fried bok choy, place the noodles in a separate medium-sized bowl, and cover them with boiling water. After 10 minutes, drain the noodles. Wilt the shredded bok choy in a separate frypan for approximately 3 minutes (you can do this while cooking the salmon patties). Serve the salmon fritters on top of the rice vermicelli and bok choy, and garnish with a dollop of mayonnaise if desired.

- For the salmon fritter burger option, warm gluten-free burger buns in the oven on high for about 5 mins. Wash and shred the lettuce. Slice the tomatoes into slices or wedges. Place the salmon fritters and salad ingredients inside the warmed gluten-free buns and add a dollop of mayonnaise for extra flavor.

Nutritional information

Calories: 628 | Fat: 22.5g | Protein: 39g | Carbs: 60.6g | Sugar: 7g

-Chapter 5-
Breakfast Recipes

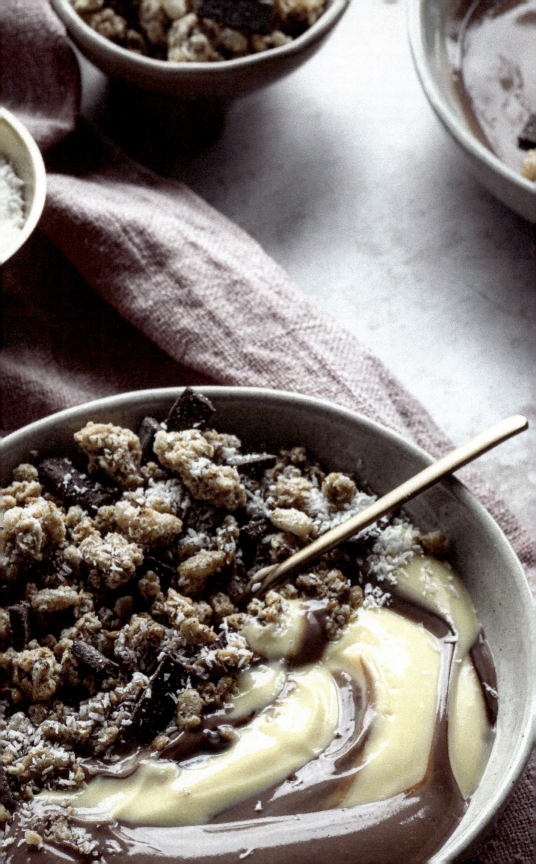

1.

Dark Chocolate Granola

Preps in 15 Min, Cooks In 40 Min, Makes 1 Serving (1/2 Cup Per Serving)

Ingredients

- 1/8 cup quinoa flakes (or rolled oats)
- 1/16 cup puffed quinoa (or puffed rice)
- 1/8 cup sunflower & pumpkin seeds (chopped)
- 1/16 cup coconut chips or dried shredded coconut
- 2/5 tbsp cocoa powder (dutch)
- 1/4 tbsp brown sugar
- 1/4 tbsp pure maple syrup
- 1/16 tsp vanilla extract
- 2/5 tbsp olive oil
- 6.25 g dark chocolate (optional, chopped into chips)
- 0 tsp sea salt (about a pinch)

Procedure

- Heat the oven to 250°F

- Combine quinoa flakes or oats, brown sugar, chopped sunflower and pumpkin seeds, coconut chips, Dutch cocoa powder, and quinoa puffs or rice bubbles in a large bowl.

- Mix olive oil, vanilla extract, and maple syrup in a separate bowl. Empty this mixture over the dry ingredients and thoroughly combine.

- Line two baking trays with baking paper then evenly spread the granola mixture. Put the trays in the heated oven and bake for 20 minutes. Afterward, gently shake or stir the granola, and continue baking for an extra 15 minutes.

- Remove the trays from the oven. Then add dark chocolate chips and a sprinkle of sea salt to taste. Return the trays to the oven and bake for another 5 minutes.

- Allow the granola to cool for 1 to 2 hours, then transfer it to airtight jars or containers for storage.

- For a delicious breakfast or snack, serve yourself 1/2 cup of granola. You can enjoy it with coconut yogurt and a serving of fresh fruit.

Nutritional information

Calories: 328 | Fat: 19.6g | Protein: 6.6g | Carbs: 22.7g | Sugar: 8.6g

Low FODMAP tips

- Ensure you opt for pure maple syrup, which is low in FOD-MAP, rather than maple-flavored syrup, as the latter may be high in FODMAP.

- Look for quinoa puffs in the gluten-free section of your nearby supermarket.

- Avoid inulin or high FODMAP sweeteners such as agave syrup, honey, high fructose, corn syrup, or fructose when selecting dark chocolate. Additionally, avoid dark chocolate varieties that include high-FODMAP fruits or nuts.

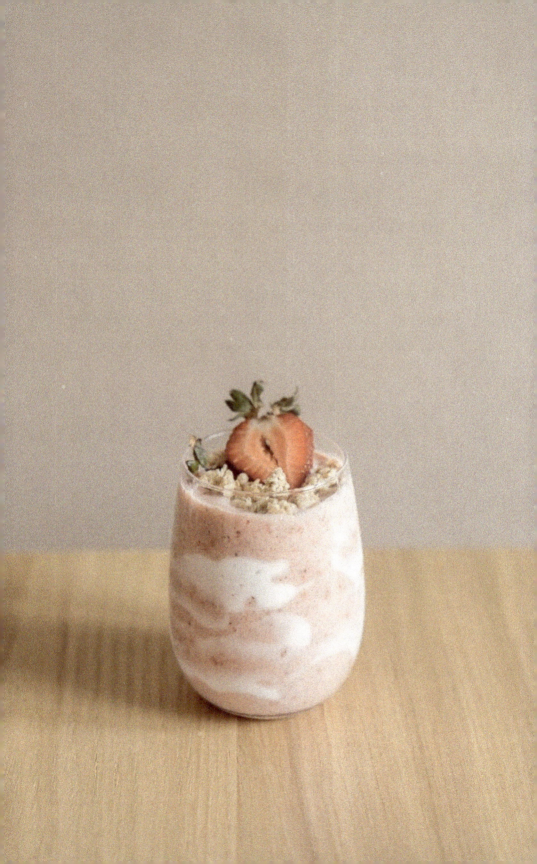

2.

Strawberry Smoothie

Preps In 5 Min, Cooks in 5 Min, Makes 1 Serving

Ingredients

- 125 ml (1/2 cup) low FODMAP milk
- 65 g strawberries (fresh or frozen)
- 60 ml (1/4 cup) vanilla soy ice cream (or lactose-free ice cream or lactose-free yoghurt)
- 1 1/2 tsp rice protein powder (optional)
- 1 tsp chia seeds
- 1/2 tbsp pure maple syrup
- 1 tsp lemon juice
- 1/4 tsp vanilla extract
- 6 ice cubes (If using fresh strawberries)

Procedure

- Depending on their size, begin by cutting the strawberries into halves or quarters.

- Combine low-FODMAP milk, strawberries, lactose-free ice cream or yogurt (such as vanilla soy ice cream or lactose-free yogurt), rice protein powder, chia seeds, maple syrup, lemon juice, and vanilla essence. Add a few ice cubes for a refreshing chill if using fresh strawberries.

- Blend the ingredients until smooth. Occasionally, the mixture may become too thick due to its cold temperature. If this happens, simply add a small amount of hot water, mix it in, and blend again.

- To fully enjoy the flavors, serving the smoothie immediately is recommended.

Nutritional information

Calories: 244 | Fat: 10.1g | Protein: 5g | Carbs: 33.5g | Sugar: 21.6g

Low FODMAP tips

- When opting for soy-based ice cream, make sure it is made from soy protein, which is low FODMAP, rather than whole soybeans, which could potentially be high FODMAP. Alternatively, you can substitute the ice cream with plain lactose-free yogurt, ensuring it doesn't contain inulin or high FODMAP sweeteners.

- Verify that your chosen low FODMAP milk does not contain high FODMAP ingredients such as agave syrup, inulin (chicory root), fructose, high fructose corn syrup, molasses, or honey.

- If selecting a dairy-free alternative, ensure that it provides 120mg of calcium per 100ml servings and 3g of protein per 100ml servings.

115

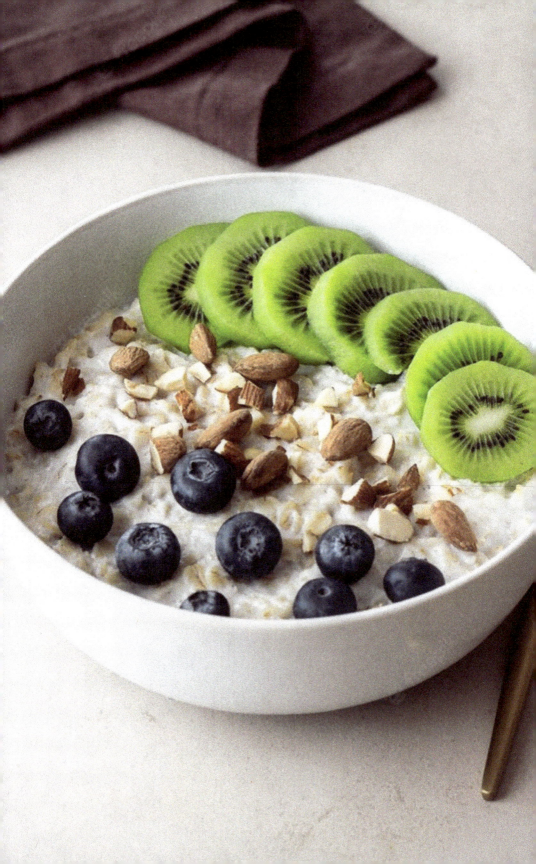

3.

Breakfast Buckwheat

Preps in 5 Min, Cooks In 10 min, Makes 1 Serving

Ingredients

- 2 cups water
- 1 cup buckwheat groats
- 1/4 cup almond milk or any alternative
- 1/4 tsp salt
- 1 tsp vanilla extract
- 1/2 tsp cinnamon

Procedure

- Start by adding water and groats in a saucepan.

- Add a pinch of a dash of cinnamon, salt, and a hint of vanilla for flavor.

- Bring the mixture to a boil and then cover the saucepan, reduce the heat to let it simmer. Allow it to simmer for 10 minutes.

- Next, stir in milk gradually and continue cooking until you achieve the desired consistency.

- Finally, feel free to personalize your dish by adding your favorite toppings. Get creative and enjoy the delicious outcome of your efforts!

Nutritional information

Calories: 221 | Fat: 2g | Protein: 8g | Carbs: 41g | Sugar: 1.6g

119

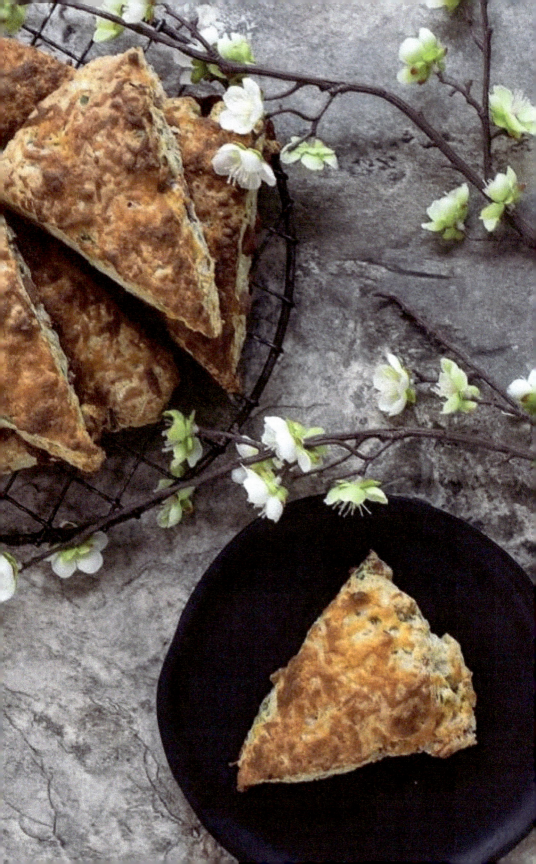

4.

Ham & Cheese Scones

Preps in 10 Min, Cooks in 18 Min, Makes 10 Servings (Serving size 1 scone)

Ingredients

- 2 1/4 cups (326 g) low FODMAP gluten-free all-purpose flour
- 1 tablespoon baking powder; use gluten-free if following a gluten-free diet
- Heaping ¼ teaspoon salt
- 1/2 cup (1 stick; 113 g) cold unsalted butter, cut into small pieces
- 1 cup (240 ml) cold lactose-free whole milk
- 1 large egg
- 4- ounces (115 g) low FODMAP diced ham
- 4- ounces (115 g) shredded cheddar cheese, divided
- 2 tablespoons finely chopped scallions, green parts

Preparation

- Heat the oven to 425°F and position the oven rack in the upper third. Prepare a half-sheet baking pan by lining it with parchment paper.

- In a bowl, whisk the baking powder, flour, and salt to aerate and combine them thoroughly.

- Add small pieces of butter to the flour mixture and use your hands to cut the butter until it resembles small raisins.

- Whisk the egg and milk till well blended in a bowl.

- Gradually drizzle the milk/egg mixture over the flour mixture while stirring and folding the ingredients together. When some flour streaks still remain, add the ham, three-quarters of the cheese, and the scallions. Continue stirring and blending until a soft dough begins to form. If the dough appears dry, use your hands to bring it together into a ball.

- Transfer the dough to the center of the prepared pan and lightly flour your hands. Pat the dough into an 8-inch round shape. Sprinkle the remaining reserved cheese evenly over the top of the scone dough, gently patting it down to help it adhere. Cut the dough into 8 wedges, divide them, and arrange them evenly spaced on the pan.

- Place the pan in the oven and bake for approximately 15 to 18 minutes. Once halfway through baking, rotate the pan to ensure even browning on the top and bottom of the scones. They should turn golden brown. Allow the pan to cool for five minutes. The scones can be served warm.

- Enjoy the scones on the day they are made for the best flavor. However, if you have leftovers, you can loosely wrap them in foil and store them at room temperature overnight. For longer storage, place the cooled scones in a heavy freezer-safe zip-top bag and freeze them for up to 1 month. When ready to consume, defrost the scones overnight in the fridge or reheat them gently in the microwave or toaster oven.

Nutritional information

Calories: 278 | Fat: 14g | Protein: 8g | Carbs: 29g | Sugar: 1g

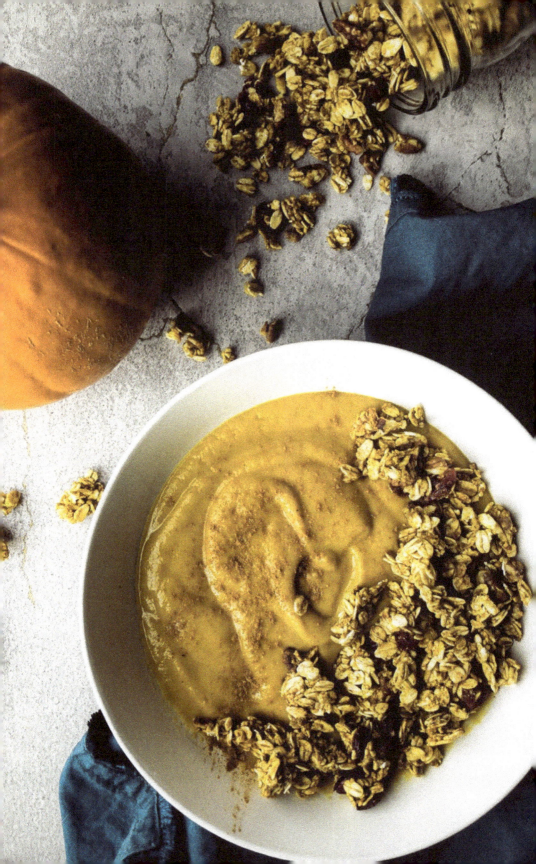

5.

Maple Pumpkin Spice Granola

Preps in 5 Min, Cooks in 40 Min, Makes 1 Serving Per Cup Cooked

Ingredients

- 3 cups (300 g) old-fashioned gluten-free rolled oats
- 3/4 cup (75 g) pecan halves
- 2 teaspoons cinnamon
- 1 teaspoon ginger
- 1/4 teaspoon nutmeg
- 1/8 teaspoon salt
- A pinch of cloves
- 1/2 cup (135 g) pure pumpkin purée
- 1/3 cup (75 ml) maple syrup
- 1/3 cup (75 ml) vegetable oil, such as canola or rice bran
- 1/4 cup (54 g) firmly packed light brown sugar
- 1 teaspoon vanilla
- 1/2 cup (80 g) dried cranberries, optional

Procedure

- Heat your oven to 325°F/165°C and position the oven rack in the middle. Prepare a rimmed baking sheet pan and set it aside.

- Combine oats, pecans, cinnamon, ginger, nutmeg, salt, and cloves in a mixing bowl. Stir them together until well combined.

- Whisk together the pumpkin purée, maple syrup, oil, vanilla, and brown sugar in a separate bowl until the mixture is smooth and thoroughly combined.

- Pour the wet mixture into the dry mixture and use a firm wooden spoon to stir everything together until well mixed. Alternatively, you can use a stand mixer by combining all the ingredients in its bowl and using a flat paddle attachment on low speed until combined.

- Scrape the mixture onto the prepared pan, spreading it out in an even layer. Bake for approximately 20 minutes. Afterward, use a large spatula to toss the granola around, ensuring that all surfaces are rotated for even baking. Continue baking for about 20 more minutes, or until the granola has just started to take on a hint of color and the delightful toasty aroma fills the air.

- Allow the pan to cool. Store the cooled granola in an airtight container at room temperature and remain fresh for up to 3 weeks.

Nutritional information

Calories: 143 | Fat: 7g | Protein: 2g | Carbs: 13g | Sugar: 5g

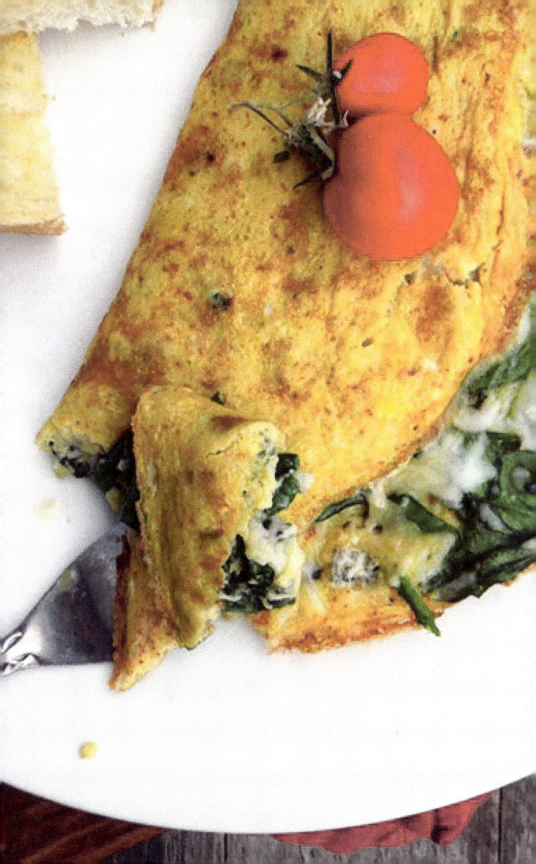

6.

BLT Omelet With Blue Cheese

Preps in 5 Min, Cooks in 5 Min, Makes 1 Serving

Ingredients

- 4 large eggs
- 2 teaspoons water
- Kosher salt
- Freshly ground black pepper
- 8 cherry or grape tomatoes, halved
- 4 pieces of cooked crisp bacon, crumbled or chopped into bite-sized pieces
- 2 ounces (55 g) crumbled blue cheese (works great with feta, too)
- Handful of baby lettuces
- 1 tablespoon unsalted butter

Preparation

- In a bowl, whisk the eggs till well beaten. Add water to the beaten eggs and season with salt and pepper. Add the tomatoes, bacon, cheese, and lettuce into the mixture, thoroughly whisking everything together.

- Heat butter in a large skillet, preferably nonstick, over low heat until it melts and becomes bubbly. Pour the omelet mixture into the skillet and cook over medium heat until the bottom begins to set. Gently use a spatula to draw in the edges of the omelet, allowing the still liquid portions to flow towards the edges and make contact with the pan. If needed, tilt the pan to assist in this process. Continue cooking until the omelet is slightly moist but not wet or overly dry.

- Once the omelet has reached the desired consistency, fold one half of it over onto the other half. Carefully put the omelet onto a plate and serve immediately while it is still hot and flavorful.

Nutritional information

Calories: 301 | Fat: 23g | Protein: 18g | Carbs: 2g | Sugar: 1g

131

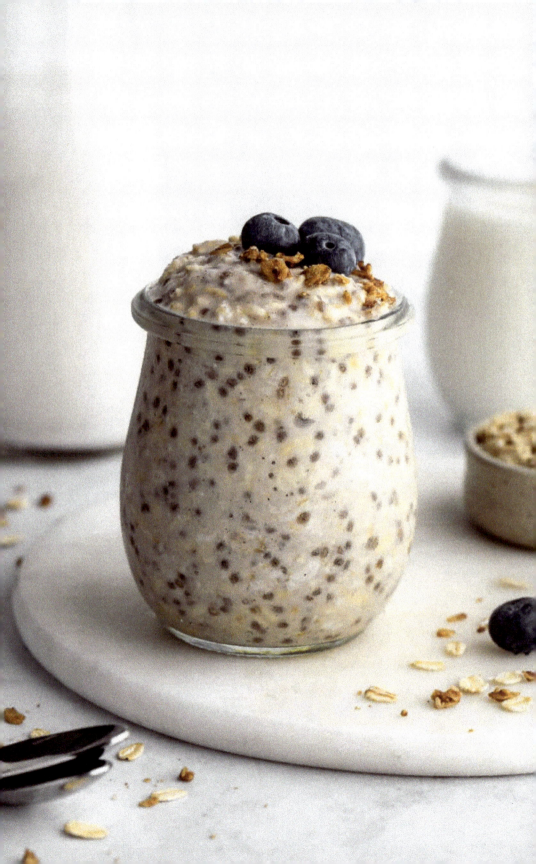

7.

Overnight Oats & Chia

Preps in 10 Min, Cooks Overnight (or for at least 8 hours), Makes 1 Serving

Ingredients

- 1 1/3 cups (315 ml) unsweetened almond milk

- 1 cup (99 g) old-fashioned rolled oats; do not use quick or instant; use gluten-free if following a gluten-free diet

- 3 tablespoons chia seeds

- 1 to 2 tablespoons maple syrup; optional

Preparation

- For convenience, combine all the ingredients in a sealed, airtight container. Shake the container vigorously to ensure everything is well combined, and then refrigerate it overnight to allow the flavors to meld.

- When ready to enjoy, simply scoop out your desired serving and heat it if desired. Add any low FODMAP toppings that suit your taste and savor the deliciousness. The mixture can be kept in the fridge for several days, making it a perfect batch to have on hand for quick and easy breakfasts or snacks throughout the week.

Nutritional information

Calories: 194 | Fat: 4g | Protein: 6g | Carbs: 31g | Sugar: 2g

-Chapter 6-

Lunch Recipes

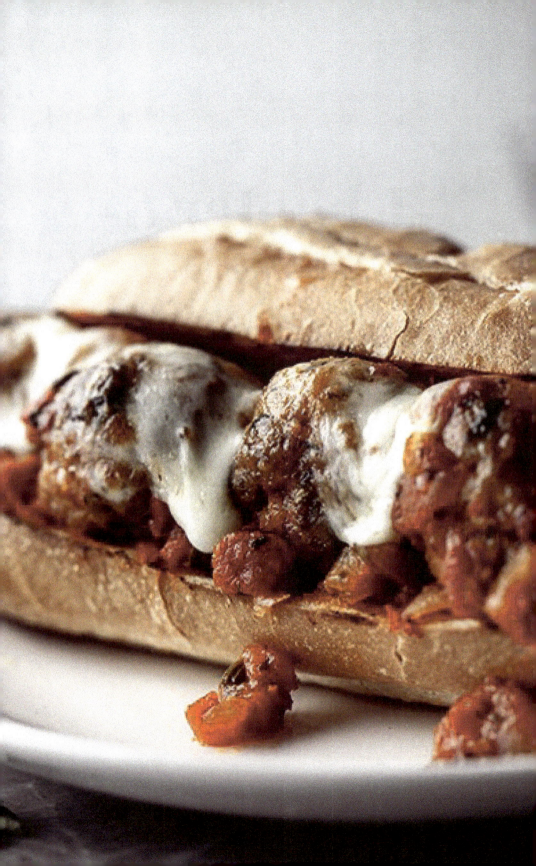

1.

Pork Meatball Subs with Sweet Red Pepper Dressing

Preps In 20 Min, Cooks In 15 Min, Makes 1 Serving

Ingredients

SWEET RED PEPPER DRESSING

- 1/8th red bell pepper
- 15 ml (1/16 cup) mayonnaise
- Season with salt & pepper

COLESLAW

- 13 g (2/5 cup) lettuce (butter, iceberg, red coral) (washed & shredded)
- 30 g (0.25 large) carrots (grated)
- 20 g (1/4 cup) common cabbage (washed & shredded)
- 2.5 g (1/16 cup) green onions/scallions (green leaves only, finely sliced)
- 1/2 tsp fresh lemon juice (couple of squeezes)
- Season with salt & pepper

PORK MEATBALLS

- 125 g lean ground pork

- 14.3 g (1/8 cup) gluten-free breadcrumbs
- 1/2 tbsp   fresh lemongrass (softcore only, finely chopped)
- 1/4 tbsp   soy sauce
- 0.25   large egg
- 1/16 tsp   dried chili flakes (optional)
- 1/2 tbsp   brown sugar
- 2.5 g (1/16 cup) green onions/scallions (green leaves only, finely sliced)

TO SERVE

- 85 g   gluten-free bread rolls
- 1 1/2 tsp   butter or dairy-free spread

Procedure

- Start by preparing the red bell pepper/capsicum. Remove the seeds and slice it into large chunks. Place the chunks on an oven tray and brush or spray them with oil. Position the tray directly under the oven grill/broiler and grill the pepper/capsicum for 5-7 minutes until the skin becomes blistered and black. Once done, remove from the oven and let it to cool.

- Next, let's make coleslaw. Cut the green leaves of the spring onion or green onion, grate the carrots, and thinly slice the cabbage and lettuce. Mix these ingredients in a bowl and season the coleslaw with a squeeze of lemon juice, a few grinds of salt, and pepper.

- Moving on to the meatballs, finely slice the green leaves of the spring onion or green onion. If using lemongrass, finely dice its soft core; otherwise, substitute with lemon juice and zest. In a large bowl, mix the pork, gluten-free breadcrumbs, lemongrass (or lemon juice and zest), chopped spring onion/green onions, soy sauce, egg, chili flakes (if desired), brown sugar, salt, and pepper until well combined. Roll the mixture into meatballs using a heaped tablespoon measure and place them on a plate.

- Cover the meatballs and microwave them for 2 minutes to ensure the center is cooked. Heat a frying pan over medium-low heat, add a splash of cooking oil, and fry the meatballs for 2-3 minutes on each side until they turn golden brown and are cooked through. You may need to cook them in two batches to ensure even cooking.

- While the meatballs are finishing, peel the roasted pepper/capsicum. Then, blend it with mayonnaise, a couple of grinds of salt, and pepper until you achieve a creamy dressing (a Nutribullet or blender can be used for this).

- Toast or heat the bread as desired.

- To assemble the subs, slice the bread and spread butter or dairy-free spread over it. Add a layer of the prepared coleslaw and top it with the cooked meatballs. Drizzle the rolls with the sweet red pepper dressing and enjoy!

Nutritional information

Calories: 370 | Fat: 16.2g | Protein: 31.9g | Carbs: 24.9g | Sugar: 9.9g

141

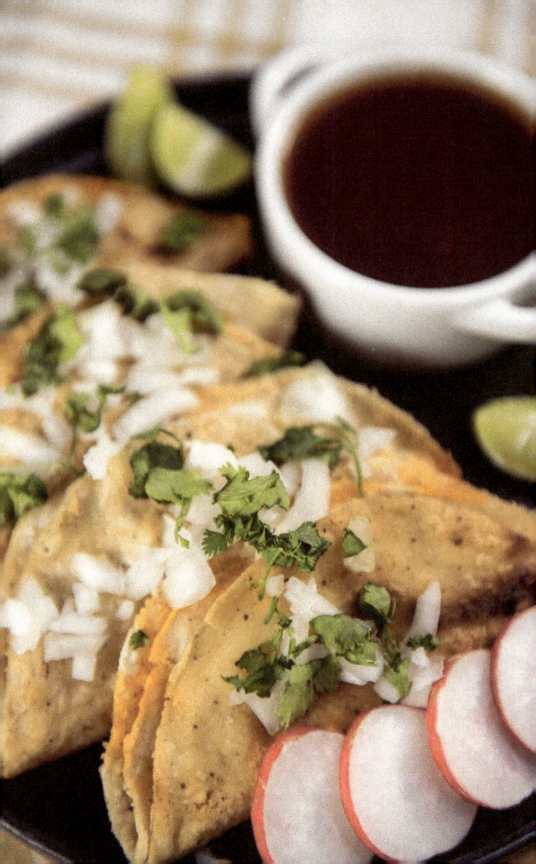

2.

Tasty Fish Bite Tortillas with Tartare Sauce

Preps In 20 Min, Cooks In 15 Min, Makes 1 Serving

Ingredients

HOMEMADE TARTARE SAUCE

- 1 tbsp   baby gherkins or cornichons (finely chopped)
- 31 ml (1/8 cup) mayonnaise
- 1/4 tsp   dried dill
- 3/4 tsp   lemon juice
- 1/8 tsp   dijon mustard
- Season with   white sugar (good pinch)
- Season with   black pepper

EASY COLESLAW

- 20 g (1/4 cup) common cabbage (washed and shredded)
- 17.5 g (1/4 cup) iceberg lettuce (washed and shredded)
- 30 g (0.5 medium) carrots (peeled and grated)
- 2.5 g (1/16 cup) green onions/scallions (green leaves only, finely sliced)
- 2/5 tsp   lemon juice (good squeeze)

- Season with salt & pepper

FISH BITES

- 125 g mild, white-fleshed fish (Cod, Haddock, Coley, Pollack, Red Snapper)
- 14.3 g (1/8 cup) gluten-free breadcrumbs
- 0.25 large egg
- 1/2 tsp Low Fodmap garlic-infused oil
- 2.5 g (1/16 cup) green onions/scallions (green leaves only, finely chopped)
- 1/2 tbsp fresh mint (finely chopped)
- 1/2 tbsp fresh parsley (finely chopped)
- 0.25 large lemon (juice and zest)
- Season with salt & pepper
- 1 tbsp neutral oil (rice bran, canola, sunflower) (for frying)

TORTILLAS

- 2 corn tortillas (for serving)

Preparation

- Start by making the homemade tartare sauce. Drain and rinse the gherkins/cornichons, then finely chop them into small pieces. In a small bowl, combine the chopped gherkins/cornichons, mayonnaise, dill, lemon juice, mustard, and a few grinds of black pepper. Mix everything till well combined. Taste the sauce and add a pinch of sugar if it's too sharp. Put the tartare sauce in the refrigerator to cool for 20 minutes before serving.

- Next, let's prepare the coleslaw. Finely shred the cabbage and lettuce, peel and grate the carrots, and thinly slice the green leaves of the spring onion/green onion. Combine the shredded cabbage, lettuce, grated carrots, and sliced spring onion/green onion in a large bowl. Squeeze a little lemon juice over the coleslaw and season with salt and pepper. Set the coleslaw aside for serving.

- Now, onto the fish bites. Cut the green leaves of the spring onion or green onion, and finely mince the mint and fresh parsley. Zest and juice the lemon. In a small bowl or glass, whisk the egg.

- Dice the fish into small pieces, ensuring they stick together without turning into a paste. Place the diced fish in a large bowl and add the sliced spring onion/green onion, mint, parsley, lemon zest, lemon juice, breadcrumbs, Low Fodmap garlic-infused oil, beaten egg, salt, and pepper. Mix everything well.

- Using a 1 tablespoon (15ml) measure, scoop the fish mixture and shape it into balls with your hands.

- Heat a frying pan over medium-low heat and add oil. Fry the fish bites in batches for about 2 minutes on each side until they turn golden and are cooked through. Adjust the heat if necessary to prevent the pan from getting too hot.

Once cooked, place the fish bites on a plate lined with paper towels to drain for a couple of minutes.

- Heat the corn tortillas according to the package instructions.

- To serve, top the tortillas with coleslaw, fish bites, and a dollop of tartare sauce. Optionally, sprinkle fresh parsley on top. Serve the remaining coleslaw on the side. Enjoy this delicious meal!

Nutritional information

Calories: 594 | Fat: 29.2g | Protein: 35g | Carbs: 50.2g | Sugar: 5.6g

147

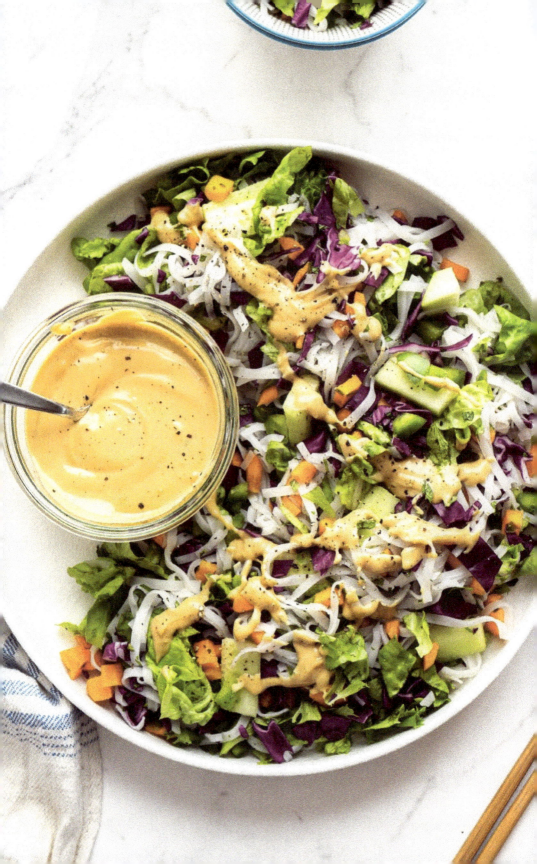

3.

Chopped Spring Roll Noodle Salad

Preps In 15 Min, Cooks In 5 Min, Makes 1 Serving

Ingredients

SALAD

- 17.5 g (1/2 cup) lettuce (butter, iceberg, red coral) (washed and shredded)
- 16.3 g (1/8 cup) green bell peppers (deseeded & diced)
- 30 g (0.25 large) carrots (peeled & grated)
- 23 g (1/4 cup) red cabbages (finely sliced)
- 1.5 g (1/16 cup) fresh mint (finely sliced)
- 30 g thin rice noodles (dry weight before cooking)
- 0.25 small cucumber (peeled & cut into small chunks)

PEANUT DRESSING

- 31 g (1/8 cup) peanut butter
- 1/4 tbsp pure maple syrup
- 1/4 tsp rice wine vinegar
- 1/2 tsp soy sauce

- 15 ml (1/16 cup) water (to thin the dressing, add more as needed)

Procedure

- Begin by cooking the rice noodles according to the instructions on the packet. Once cooked, drain the noodles, rinse them under cold water, and drain again. Set them aside for later use.

- Prepare the salad ingredients by washing and shredding the lettuce, dicing the green bell pepper/capsicum, peeling, and dicing the carrot, shredding the cabbage, and slicing the cucumber into bite-sized pieces. Finely chop the mint. Mix all the salad ingredients in a bowl.

- Now, let's make the peanut dressing. Whisk together the peanut butter, maple syrup, rice wine vinegar, soy sauce, and water in a bowl till well combined. Alternatively, you can use a blender. Add more water to thin the dressing to your desired consistency if needed.

- If the rice noodles are too long, you can cut them in half using scissors.

- Add the rice noodles to the salad bowl and toss everything together to combine. Drizzle the peanut dressing over the salad and mix well to ensure all the ingredients are coated.

- If you plan to meal prep, this salad can be kept in the refrigerator for up to 3 days. We recommend storing the dressing separately and adding it to the salad before serving. Enjoy this refreshing and flavorful salad!

Nutritional information

Calories: 343 | Fat: 16.5g | Protein: 10.3g | Carbs: 41.8g | Sugar: 9.8g

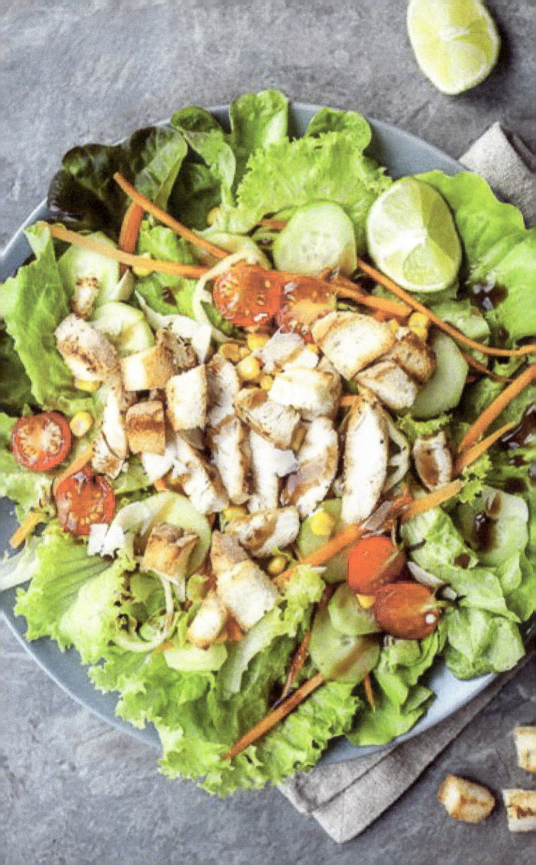

4.

Grilled Chicken Salad

Preps in 10 Min, Cooks in 15 Min, Makes 2 Servings

Ingredients

- 2 boneless, skinless chicken breasts
- Mixed salad greens
- 1 cucumber, sliced
- 2 tomatoes, diced
- 1 carrot, shredded
- 2 tablespoons olive oil
- 1 tablespoon lemon juice
- Salt and pepper to taste

Procedure

- Preheat the grill to medium heat.
- Season the chicken breasts with salt and pepper.
- Grill the chicken for about 6-8 minutes per side until cooked through.
- Let the chicken rest for a few minutes, then slice it into strips.
- Combine the salad greens, cucumber, tomatoes, and carrot in a bowl.

- Whisk the olive oil and lemon juice in a bowl to make the dressing.
- Add the sliced chicken to the salad and drizzle with the dressing.
- Toss gently to combine and serve.

Nutritional information

Calories: 300 | Fat: 15g | Protein: 30g | Carbs: 10g

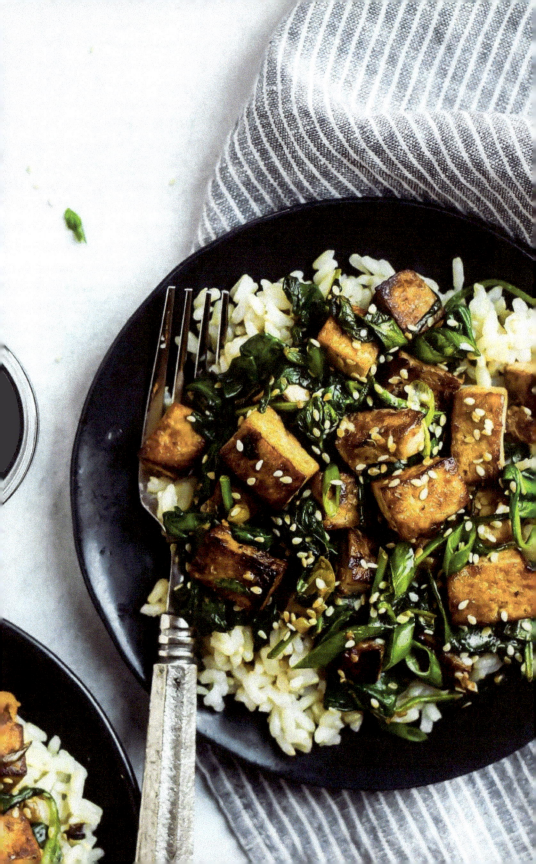

5.

Tofu Stir-Fry

Preps in 15 Min, Cooks in 10 Min, Makes 2 Servings

Ingredients

- 1 block firm tofu, drained and cubed
- 1 cup sliced zucchini
- 1 cup sliced bell peppers (any color)
- 1 cup sliced carrots
- 1 cup bok choy, chopped
- 2 tablespoons gluten-free soy sauce
- 1 tablespoon rice vinegar
- 1 tablespoon sesame oil
- 1 teaspoon grated ginger
- 2 green onions, sliced (the white part is high in FODMAP, so avoid them)
- Salt and pepper to taste

Procedure

- Heat the sesame oil in a pan over medium-low heat.
- Add the tofu cubes and cook until browned on all sides, about 5 minutes. Remove from the skillet and set aside.

- Add the zucchini, bell peppers, carrots, and bok choy in the same skillet. Stir-fry for about 5 minutes until the vegetables are tender-crisp.
- Whisk together the gluten-free soy sauce, rice vinegar, grated ginger, and green onions in a bowl.
- Return the tofu to the skillet and pour the sauce over the tofu and vegetables.
- Stir-fry for another 2 minutes to heat through.
- Season with salt and pepper to taste and then serve.

Nutritional information

Calories: 250 | Fat: 10g | Protein: 15g | Carbs: 30g

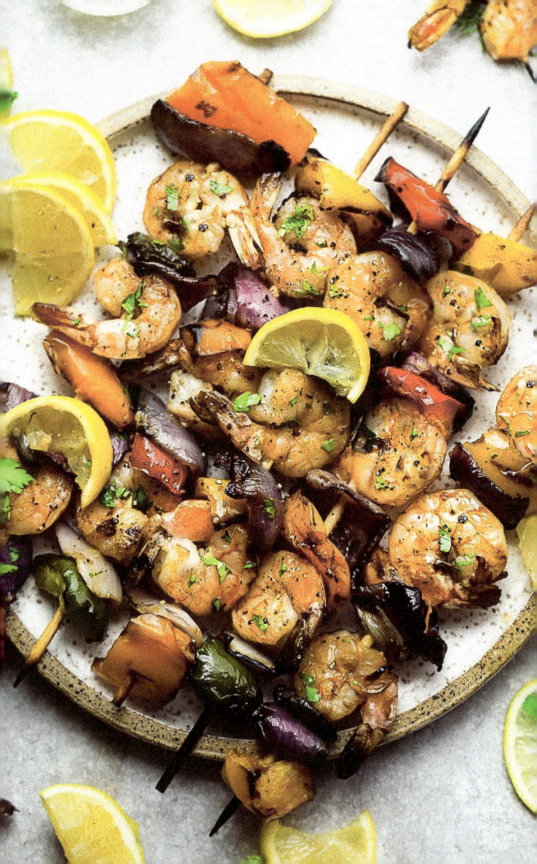

6.

Shrimp and Vegetable Skewers

Preps in 20 Min, Cooks in 10 Min, Makes 6 Servings

Ingredients

- 1 pound shrimp, peeled and deveined
- 1 zucchini, cut into chunks
- 1 small eggplant, cut into chunks
- 2 tablespoons olive oil
- 1 bell pepper (any color), cut into chunks
- 2 tablespoons fresh lemon juice
- 1 tablespoon chopped fresh herbs (such as basil or parsley)
- Salt and pepper to taste

Procedure

- Heat the grill or grill pan to medium-low heat.
- Thread the shrimp, zucchini, bell pepper, and eggplant onto skewers, alternating between ingredients.
- Whisk the olive oil, lemon juice, fresh herbs, salt, and pepper in a bowl.
- Brush the skewers with the olive oil mixture.
- Grill the skewers for 3-4 minutes per side until the shrimp is cooked and the vegetables are tender.

- Remove from the grill and serve hot.

Nutritional information

Calories: 200 | Fat: 8g | Protein: 20g | Carbs: 10g

163

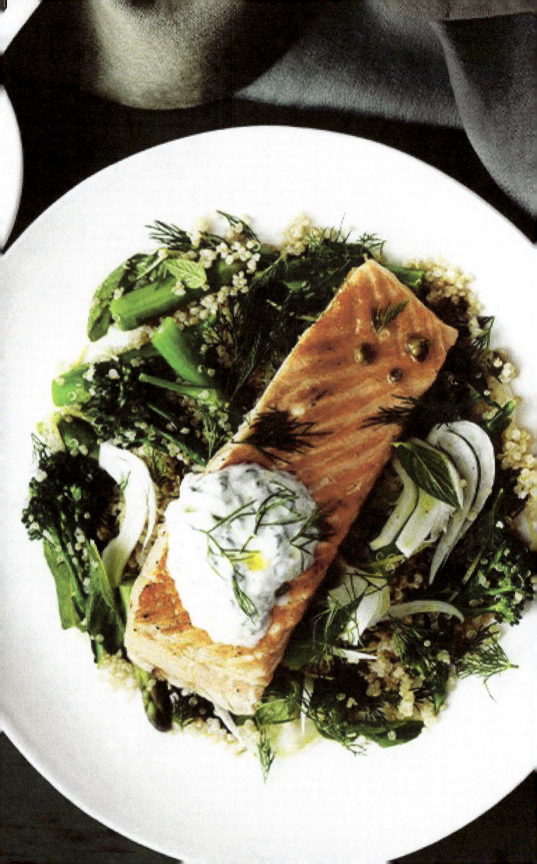

7.

Salmon and Quinoa Bowl

Preps in 10 Min, Cooks in 20 Min, Makes 2 Servings

Ingredients

- 2 salmon fillets
- 1/2 cup sliced bell peppers (any color)
- 1 cup cooked quinoa
- 1 cup steamed broccoli florets
- 2 tablespoons gluten-free soy sauce
- 1 tablespoon sesame oil
- 1 tablespoon sesame seeds
- Salt and pepper to taste

Procedure

- Heat the oven to 400°F
- Put the salmon fillets on a baking sheet and season with salt and pepper.
- Bake for about 12-15 minutes until the salmon is cooked through.
- Combine the cooked quinoa, steamed broccoli, and sliced bell peppers in a large bowl.

- Whisk together the gluten-free soy sauce, sesame oil, and sesame seeds to make the dressing in a small bowl.
- Add the baked salmon to the bowl and drizzle with the dressing.
- Toss gently to combine and serve.

Nutritional information

Calories: 400 | Fat: 20g | Protein: 30g | Carbs: 25g

-Chapter 7-
Dinner Recipes

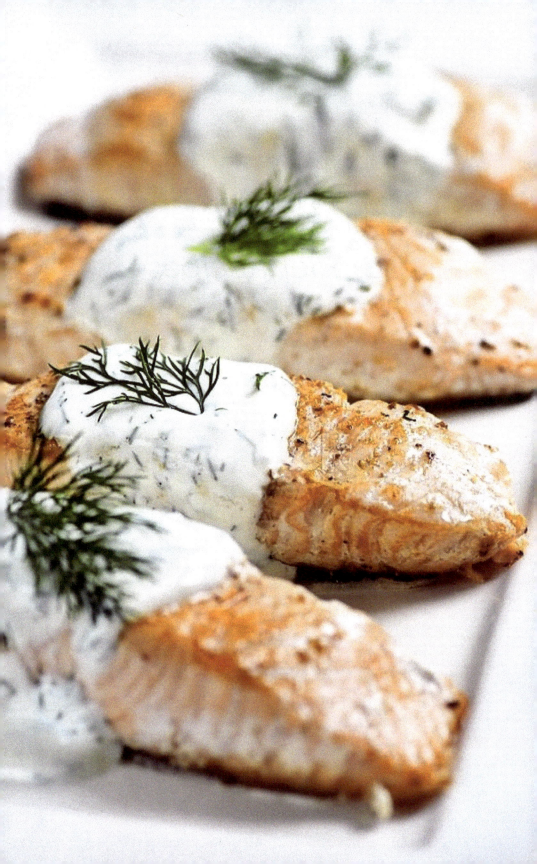

1.

Baked Salmon with Dill Sauce

Preps in 10 Min, Cooks in 20 Min, Makes 4 Servings

Ingredients

- 4 salmon fillets
- 2 tablespoons olive oil
- Salt and pepper to taste
- 1 tablespoon fresh dill, chopped
- 1/2 cup lactose-free yogurt
- 1 tablespoon lemon juice

Procedure

- Preheat the oven to 375°F.
- Place the salmon fillets on a baking sheet lined with parchment paper.
- Drizzle the salmon with olive oil. Season with salt, pepper, and fresh dill.
- Bake for about 15-20 mins, or till the salmon is cooked and breaks easily with a fork.
- Meanwhile, in a small bowl, mix the lactose-free yogurt and lemon juice to make the dill sauce.

- Serve the baked salmon with the dill sauce on the side.

Nutritional Information

Calories: 350 | Fat: 25g | Protein: 25g | Carbs: 2g

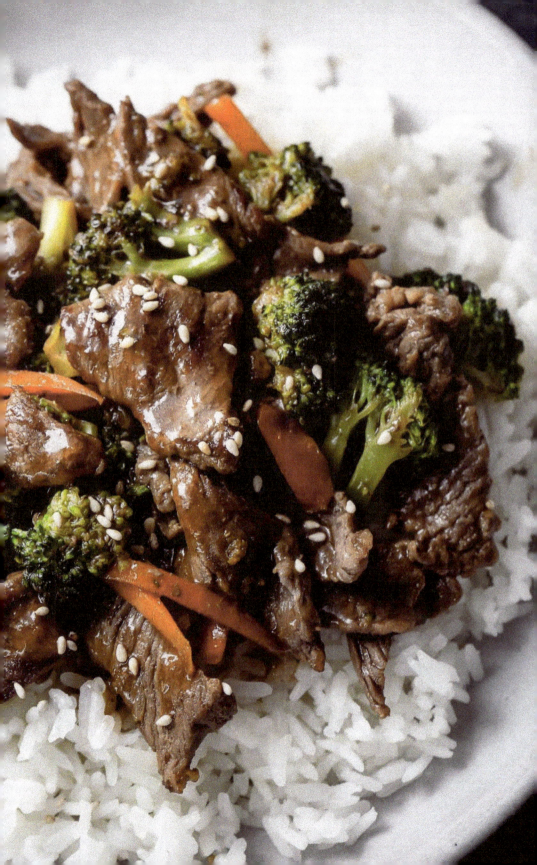

2.

Beef and Broccoli Stir-Fry

Preps in 15 Min, Cooks in 15 Min, Makes 4 Servings

Ingredients

- 1 lb (450g) beef sirloin, thinly sliced
- 2 tablespoons low FODMAP soy sauce
- 1 tablespoon sesame oil
- 1 tablespoon grated fresh ginger
- 2 tablespoons Low Fodmap garlic-infused oil
- 4 cups broccoli florets
- 2 medium carrots, thinly sliced
- 1/2 cup low FODMAP beef broth
- 1 tablespoon cornstarch (optional for thickening)

Procedure

- Combine the sliced beef with the low FODMAP soy sauce, sesame oil, and grated ginger in a bowl. Set aside to marinate for 10 minutes.

- Heat the Low Fodmap garlic-infused oil in a skillet or wok over medium-high heat. Add the beef and stir-fry for 3-4 mins until browned. Remove the beef from the skillet and put it aside.

- Add the broccoli florets, carrots, and beef broth in the same skillet. Stir-fry for about 5-6 minutes until the vegetables are crisp-tender.

- If desired, mix the cornstarch with a little water to make a slurry and add it to the skillet to thicken the sauce. Stir until the sauce thickens.

- Return the cooked beef to the skillet and toss to coat everything in the sauce.

- Serve hot with rice or quinoa, if desired.

Nutritional Information

Calories: 280 | Fat: 15g | Protein: 25g | Carbs: 10g

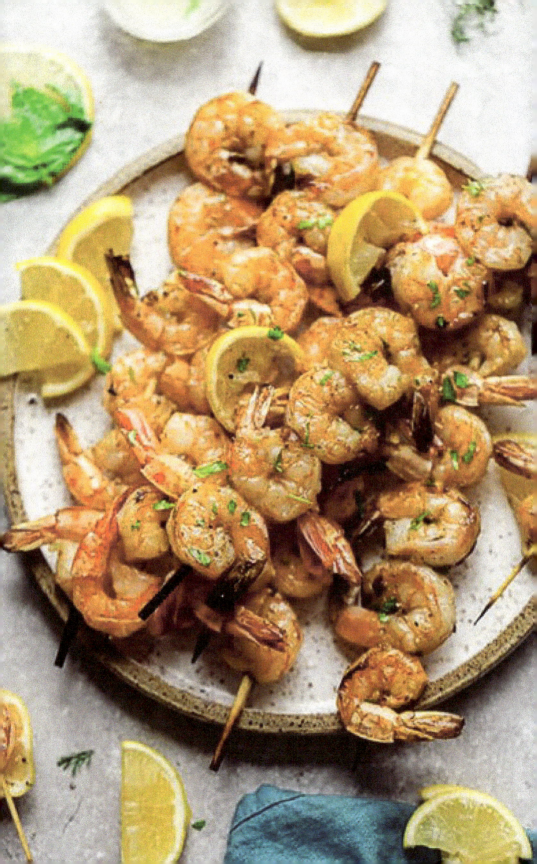

3.

Lemon Herb Shrimp Skewers

Preps in 15 Min, Cooks in 10 Min, Makes 4 Servings

Ingredients

- 1 lb (450g) shrimp, peeled and deveined
- 2 tablespoons olive oil
- 2 tablespoons fresh parsley, chopped
- 1 tablespoon fresh thyme, chopped
- 2 lemons, juiced and zested
- Salt and pepper to taste

Procedure

- Heat the grill to medium-high heat.
- Combine the olive oil, parsley, thyme, lemon zest, lemon juice, salt, and pepper in a bowl.
- Thread the shrimp onto skewers and brush them with the lemon and herb mixture.
- Grill the shrimp skewers on each side for about 2-3 minutes until they turn pink and opaque.
- Serve hot with a side of low-FODMAP salad or roasted vegetables.

Nutritional Information

Calories: 180 | Fat: 8g | Protein: 25g | Carbs: 3g

179

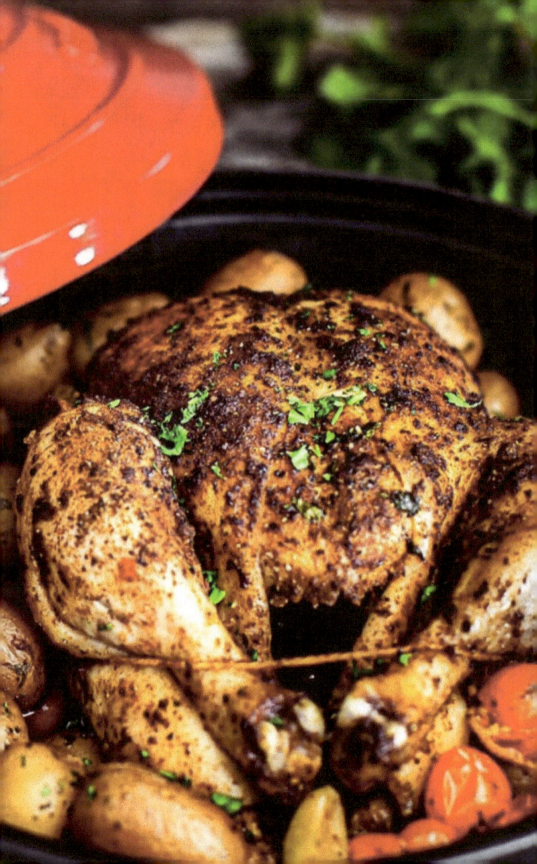

4.

Moroccan Spiced Roasted Chicken Thighs

Preps in 10 Min, Cooks in 35 Min, Makes 4 Servings

Ingredients

- 8 bone-in, skin-on chicken thighs
- 2 tablespoons olive oil
- 2 teaspoons ground cumin
- 1 teaspoon ground coriander
- 1 teaspoon ground paprika
- 1/2 teaspoon ground cinnamon
- Salt and pepper to taste
- Fresh cilantro for garnish

Procedure

- Preheat the oven to 400°F.
- Put the chicken thighs on a baking sheet lined with parchment paper.
- In a small bowl, combine the olive oil, cumin, coriander, paprika, cinnamon, salt, and pepper. Mix well.
- Brush the chicken thighs with the spice mixture, coat them evenly.

- Roast in the oven for 30 to 35 minutes or till the chicken is cooked and the skin is crunchy.
- Garnish with fresh cilantro and serve with a side of low-FODMAP roasted vegetables or a green salad.

Nutritional Information

Calories: 380 | Fat: 30g | Protein: 25g | Carbs: 1g

183

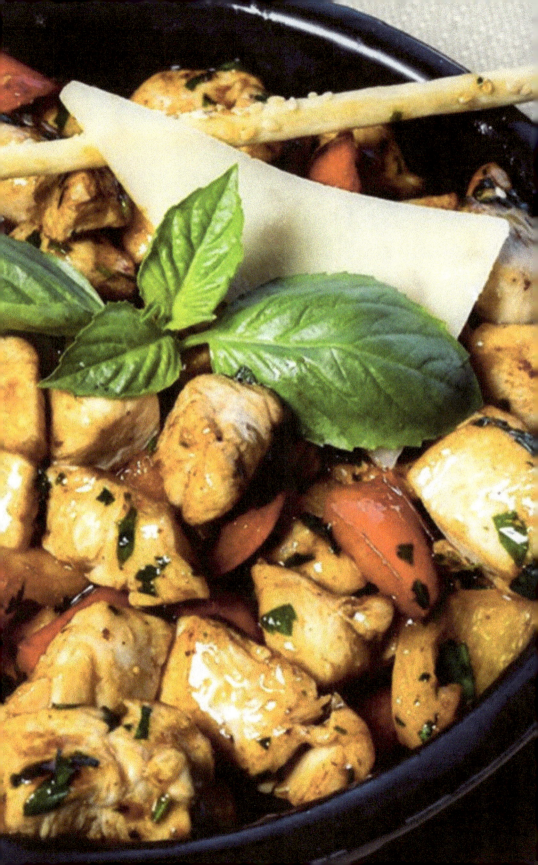

5.

Tofu and Vegetable Curry

Preps in 15 Min, Cooks in 25 Min, Makes 4 Servings

Ingredients

- 1 package (14 oz or 400g) of firm tofu, drained and cubed
- 2 tablespoons Low Fodmap garlic-infused oil
- 1 tablespoon grated fresh ginger
- 1 red bell pepper, thinly sliced
- 1 zucchini, diced
- 1 cup canned diced tomatoes
- 1 cup low FODMAP vegetable broth
- 2 tablespoons low FODMAP curry powder
- 1/2 cup lactose-free coconut milk
- Salt and pepper to taste
- Fresh cilantro for garnish

Procedure

- Heat the Low Fodmap garlic-infused oil in a skillet or wok over medium-high heat. Add the tofu cubes and cook till golden brown on all sides. Remove the tofu from the skillet and set aside.

- Add the grated ginger, red bell pepper, and zucchini in the same skillet. Stir-fry for about 3-4 minutes until the vegetables start to soften.
- Add the diced tomatoes, vegetable broth, curry powder, and cooked tofu to the skillet. Stir to combine.
- Reduce heat to low and simmer for about 15 minutes, until the flavors are well combined, and the vegetables are tender.
- Stir in the lactose-free coconut milk and season with salt and pepper. Simmer for an additional 5 minutes.
- Garnish with fresh cilantro and serve hot with rice or quinoa.

Nutritional Information

Calories: 280 | Fat: 15g | Protein: 15g | Carbs: 15g

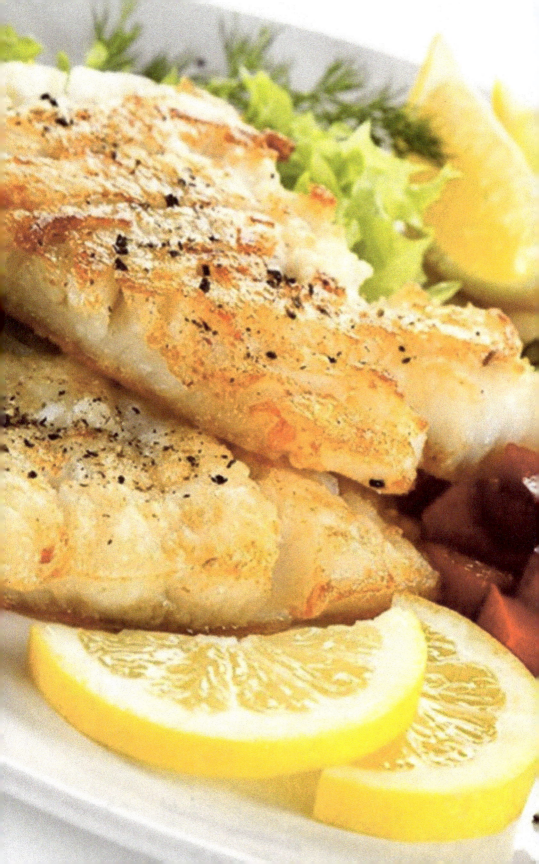

6.

Baked Cod with Lemon and Dill

Preps in 10 Min, Cooks in 15 Min, Makes 4 Servings

Ingredients

- 4 cod fillets
- 2 tablespoons olive oil
- 2 tablespoons fresh dill, chopped
- 1 lemon, juiced and zested
- Salt and pepper to taste

Procedure

- Preheat the oven to 400°F. Put the cod fillets on a baking sheet lined with parchment paper.
- Drizzle the cod with olive oil and season with salt, pepper, fresh dill, lemon juice, and lemon zest.
- Bake for about 12-15 minutes until the cod is opaque and breaks easily with a fork.
- Serve hot with a side of low-FODMAP roasted potatoes or steamed vegetables.

Nutritional Information

Calories: 200 | Fat: 10g | Protein: 25g | Carbs: 1g

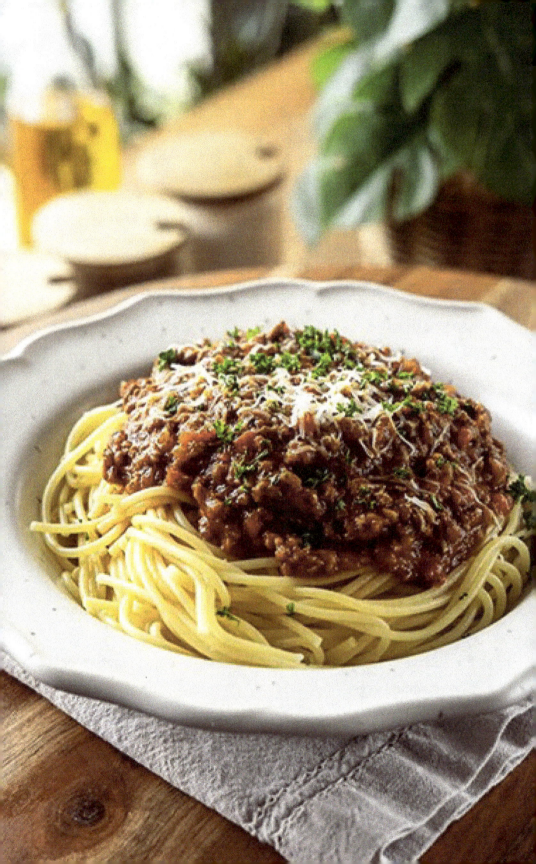

7.

Spaghetti with Meat Sauce

Preps in 10 Min, Cooks in 30 Min, Makes 4 Servings

Ingredients

- 8 ounces of gluten-free spaghetti
- 1 pound ground beef
- 1 tablespoon Low Fodmap garlic-infused olive oil
- 1 cup canned tomato sauce
- 1 cup canned diced tomatoes
- 1 tablespoon tomato paste
- 1 teaspoon dried oregano
- 1 teaspoon dried basil
- Salt and pepper to taste
- Fresh parsley, chopped (for garnish)

Procedure

- Cook gluten-free spaghetti. Follow the instructions on the packaging
- Drain and set aside.
- In a large skillet, heat the Low Fodmap garlic-infused olive oil over medium heat.

- Add the ground beef and cook till browned and cooked through.
- Stir in the tomato sauce, diced tomatoes, tomato paste, dried oregano, dried basil, salt, and pepper.
- Simmer the sauce for 10-15 minutes, allowing the flavors to meld together.
- Serve the meat sauce over the cooked gluten-free spaghetti.
- Garnish with fresh parsley.

Nutritional Information

Calories: 460 | Fat: 12g | Protein: 26g | Carbs: 62g

Conclusion

As you reach the final pages of the Low FODMAP Diet, you find yourself at the culmination of a transformative journey. This book has empowered you to take charge of your digestive health, embrace mindful eating, and discover the incredible power of food as medicine.

From the beginning, my goal was clear—to provide a collection of delicious and nutritious recipes that would not only adhere to the dietary restrictions of the Low FODMAP Diet but also ignite a passion for flavorful and enjoyable eating.

Throughout the pages of this cookbook, you have explored the intricate world of FODMAPs, those fermentable carbohydrates that can cause discomfort and digestive distress. You have learned to identify high FODMAP foods and understand the importance of following a low FODMAP diet to alleviate symptoms such as bloating, gas, and abdominal pain. Armed with this knowledge, you have opened a realm of possibilities where food can be both kind to our bodies and a source of pleasure.

From breakfast to dinner, this book proves that a low FODMAP diet does not mean sacrificing flavor or variety. You have embraced the abundance of fruits and vegetables within the low

FODMAP spectrum and learned to create mouthwatering dishes that showcase their natural goodness. You have experimented with herbs, spices, and condiments that add depth and complexity to your meals without causing digestive distress. And most importantly, you have celebrated the joy of cooking and eating, finding delight in each bite.

But this book is more than just a collection of recipes. It's a resource that has provided essential tips and tricks for successful meal preparation, guidance on managing dining out and social gatherings while following the diet, and valuable insights into maintaining a balanced and nourishing diet beyond FODMAPs.

As you close this chapter of your journey, remember that the Low FODMAP Diet is not a one-size-fits-all solution. It is a framework that can be tailored to your unique needs and preferences. Experiment with the recipes, modify ingredients to suit your taste and don't be afraid to explore new flavors and combinations.

Always listen to your body and its reactions. Take note of how different foods make you feel and make adjustments accordingly. Remember, the ultimate goal is to eliminate trigger foods and create a sustainable and enjoyable eating pattern that supports your well-being.

I hope that this cookbook has provided you with inspiration, knowledge, and a sense of empowerment. May it serve as a faithful companion on your continued journey toward a healthier and happier you. Embrace the joy of cooking, savor each bite, and nourish your body with the abundance of flavors that await you.

Bon appétit and bon voyage on your ongoing Low FODMAP adventure!

Thank You

Thank you so much for purchasing my book.

You could have picked from dozens of other books, but you took a chance and chose this one.

So, THANK YOU for getting this book and for making it all the way to the end.

Before you go, I wanted to ask you for one small favor. **Could you please consider posting a review on the platform? Posting a review is the best and easiest way to support the work of independent authors like me.**

Your feedback will help me to keep writing the kind of books that will help you get the results you want. It would mean a lot to me to hear from you.

Resources

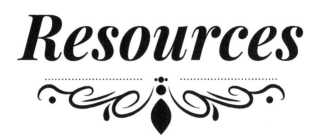

https://www.nhs.uk/conditions/irritable-bowel-syndrome-ibs/#:~:text=The%20exact%20cause%20is%20unknown,a%20family%20history%20of%20IBS.

https://www.ncbi.nlm.nih.gov/pmc/articles/PMC7019579/

https://pubmed.ncbi.nlm.nih.gov/28244669/

https://www.ncbi.nlm.nih.gov/pmc/articles/PMC5372955/

https://www.ncbi.nlm.nih.gov/pmc/articles/PMC7019579/

https://www.ncbi.nlm.nih.gov/pubmed/25982757

https://www.ncbi.nlm.nih.gov/pmc/articles/PMC7019579/

https://www.ncbi.nlm.nih.gov/pubmed/17490952

https://go.skimresources.com/?id=71026X1587439&isjs=1&jv=15.3.0-stackpath&sref=https%3A%2F%2Fwww.bbcgoodfood.com%2Fhowto%2Fguide%2Fhow-does-diet-affect-gut-health&url=https%3A%2F%2Fpubmed.ncbi.nlm.nih.gov%2F32612660%2F&xs=1&xtz=0&xuuid=e8fa059b9b9b5b25f5b43dfc3c67f189&xcust=bbcgoodfood-289354&xjsf=other_click__auxclick%20%5B2%5D

https://go.skimresources.com/?id=71026X1587439&isjs=1&jv=15.3.0-stack-

path&sref=https%3A%2F%2Fwww.bbcgood-food.com%2Fhowto%2Fguide%2Fhow-does-diet-affect-gut-health&url=https%3A%2F%2Fwww.ncbi.nlm.nih.gov%2Fpmc%2Farti-cles%2FPMC3426293%2F&xs=1&xtz=0&xuuid=e8fa059b9b9b5b25f5b43dfc3c67f189&xcust=bbcgoodfood-289354&xjsf=other_click__auxclick%20%5B2%5D

https://link.springer.com/article/10.1007/s11894-013-0370-0

https://www.uofmhealth.org/health-library/uf4696

https://www.ncbi.nlm.nih.gov/pmc/articles/PMC2892765/

https://doi.org/10.3892/ijmm.2017.3072

Your Free Gift

As a way of saying thanks for your purchase, I'm offering a copy of our **Digestive Health Wellness Guide**: *The Ultimate Digestive Health Wellness Guide To Understanding Your Gut And Living A More Pain-Free Life* for FREE to you!

To get instant access just go to: **prestigebookgroup.com**

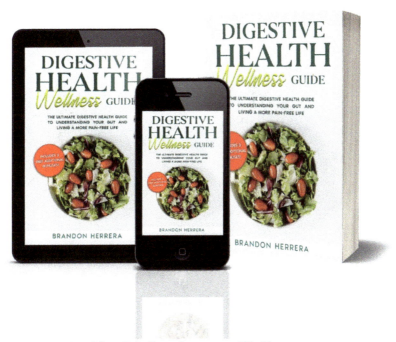

Inside this book you will discover:

- **14 Simple Tips** to improving your digestive health today
- How to prioritize these **4 mealtime habits** to get your digestive process working properly

- 5 of the most common forms of digestive health issues
- A quick gut health food checklist that *all dietitians* swear by
- And so much more!

If you want to conquer digestive health and live a more pain-free life, make sure to grab this free guide.

Printed in the USA
CPSIA information can be obtained
at www.ICGtesting.com
LVHW010739210923
758625LV00005B/69